SLEEP MEDICINE SECRETS

SLEEP MEDICINE SECRETS

DAMIEN STEVENS, MD
Assistant Professor of Medicine and Psychology
Sleep Disorder Service and Research Center
Rush University Medical Center
Chicago, Illinois

HANLEY & BELFUS, INC.
An Imprint of Elsevier

BS

HANLEY & BELFUS, INC.
An Imprint of Elsevier

The Curtis Center
Independence Square West
Philadelphia, Pennsylvania 19106

Note to the reader: Although the information in this book has been carefully reviewed for accuracy, neither the authors nor the editor nor the publisher can accept any legal responsibility for any errors or omissions that may be made. Neither the publisher nor the editor makes any warranty, expressed or implied, with respect to the material contained herein.

Library of Congress Control Number: 2004103675

SLEEP MEDICINE SECRETS   1-56053-592-X

Printed in the United States

Last digit is the print number: 9 8 7 6 5 4 3 2 1

5/12/06

TABLE OF CONTENTS

CONTRIBUTORS

Rosalind Cartwright, PhD
Professor and Chairman, Department of Psychology, Rush University Medical Center, Affiliated Scientist, Rush-Presbyterian-St. Luke's Hospital, Chicago, Illinois

Glenn A. Clark, RPSGT
Polysomnographic Technologist, Sleep Disorders Service and Research Center, Rush University Medical Center, Chicago, Illinois

Flavia B. Consens, MD
Assistant Professor, Neurology, University of Michigan, Associate Director, Sleep Disorders Center, Ann Arbor, Michigan

James M. Cygan, MD
Medical Director, Watson Hospital Sleep Disorder Center, Pulmonary and Critical Care Consultants, Watson, Wisconsin

James J. Herdegen, MD
Assistant Professor, Internal Medicine, Section of Pulmonary and Critical Care, Rush University Medical Center, Rush Medical Center, Chicago, Illinois

Lisa J. Meltzer, PhD
Pickwick Fellow, Children's Hospital of Philadelphia, Philadelphia, Pennsylvania

Jodi A. Mindell, PhD
Professor, Psychology, St. Joseph's University, Children's Hospital of Philadelphia, Philadelphia, Pennsylvania

Babak Mokhlesi, MD
Assistant Professor of Medicine, Division of Pulmonary and Critical Care Medicine, Rush University Medical School, Director of the Sleep Laboratory at Cook County Hospital, Chicago, Illinois

Jean M. Silvestri, MD
Associate Professor of Pediatrics, Pediatrics, Rush Medical College of Rush University, Rush Children's Hospital, Rush University Medical Center, Chicago, Illinois

Mark L. Splaingard, MD
Professor of Clinical Pediatrics, Ohio State University, Columbus Children's Hospital, Columbus, Ohio

Edward J. Stephanski, PhD
Associate Professor of Psychology and Medicine, Department of Psychology, Rush Medical College, Director, Sleep Disorders Service and Research Center, Rush University Medical Center, Chicago, Illinois

Suzanne Stevens, MD, MS
Assistant Professor, Neurology and Psychology, Rush University Medical Center, Chicago, Illinois

Aiman Tulaimat, MD
Assistant Professor of Medicine, Divisions of Pulmonary and Critical Care Medicine, Rush University Medical Center, John H. Stroger Jr. Hospital at Cook County, Chicago, Illinois

Debra E. Weese-Mayer, MD
Professor of Pediatrics, Rush University, Director, Pediatric Respiratory Medicine, Rush University Medical Center, Chicago, Illinois

James K. Wyatt, PhD
Assistant Professor of Psychology, Department of Psychology, Rush Medical College, Laboratory Director, Sleep Disorders Center, Rush University Medical Center, Chicago, Illinois

PREFACE

It is with great pleasure to present to you this book in its completed form. I am sincerely grateful to all contributing authors who made this book a reality. My intent in compiling *Sleep Medicine Secrets* was many-fold, but the main goal was to produce an inexpensive introductory text for people interested in the field of sleep medicine. The book is geared toward a wide audience, from medical students to clinicians practicing sleep medicine. The chapters cover basic science, neurophysiology and clinical aspects of sleep. It must be stressed that this book is not meant to be a comprehensive reference.

I would like to dedicate this book to my two year old son and newborn daughter . . . may they both master the art of sleep soon. Finally, I must thank my most patient and understanding wife, without whom this text would never have been completed.

Damien Stevens, MD

TOP SECRETS

These 100 secrets summarize the concepts, principles, and most salient details relevant to sleep medicine.

1. Sleep is defined behaviorally as a reversible unconscious state with characteristic supine sleep posture, lack of mobility, closed eyes, and increased arousal threshold.

2. Sleep is divided into non–rapid-eye-movement (NREM) sleep and rapid-eye-movement (REM) sleep.

3. NREM sleep is further divided into four stages (stages I–IV) based on the electroencephalogram (EEG). REM sleep is divided based on the absence or presence of short-lived bursts of eye movement into two types, tonic REM and phasic REM, respectively.

4. The sleep period, the time from sleep onset at night until awakening in the morning, does not change with age, but total sleep time, the sleep period minus the duration of awakenings, commonly decreases in aging adults. Many older adults compensate by napping during the day.

5. The most common changes in sleep architecture related to aging include a reduction in duration and voltage of SWS, an increase in the number and duration of nocturnal arousals and awakenings, and a slight reduction in REM sleep.

6. Sympathetic tone is typically decreased during NREM sleep, but during arousals sympathetic tone usually increases in bursts of activity.

7. Systemic blood pressure falls during NREM sleep by approximately 10%, but during REM sleep blood pressure fluctuates significantly.

8. Because NREM sleep leads to a decline in heart rate, mean arterial pressure, and sympathetic nerve activity, sleep represents a state of cardiovascular quiescence with reduced myocardial workload.

9. During tonic REM sleep, parasympathetic tone is increased while sympathetic tone reaches it lowest level. However, during phasic REM periods, sympathetic activity transiently increases with an associated increased in mean arterial pressure and heart rate.

10. Prolactin is one of the hormones most strongly influenced by sleep with a nearly flat curve after sleep restriction, whereas cortisol secretion shows minimal influence with essentially the same secretion even with sleep deprivation.

11. Growth hormone shows pulsatile secretions during slow-wave sleep that is suppressed during sleep restriction.

12. Norepinephrine, dopamine, acetylcholine, histamine, and glutamate are the major neurotransmitters that are thought to promote wakefulness; serotonin, adenosine, and gamma-amino butyric acid (GABA) are thought to promote sleep.

13. The suprachiasmatic nucleus (SCN) is composed of paired nuclei located in the anterior hypothalamus, dorsal to the optic chiasm. The retinohypothalamic tract sends input directly to the SCN to help modulate circadian rhythms.

14. Hypocretins are proteins that regulate wakefulness and sleep. Narcopelopsy is associated with a lack of neurons responsible for making hypocretin, and studies of cerebrospinal fluid (CSF) have shown absent or extremely low levels of hypocretin in patients with narcolepsy.

15. The initial REM period occurs at the end of the first sleep cycle, at approximately 70-120 minutes after sleep onset, depending on age and other factors. The REM periods usually progressively increase in length, and 4–6 REM periods are typically seen across the course of the night.

16. A shortened REM latency can be seen with depression, narcolepsy, and withdrawal of REM-suppressing medications such as antidepressants or alcohol. In addition, REM latency may be short during recovery sleep, as sometimes seen during titration of continuous positive airway pressure (CPAP).

17. Slow-wave sleep is more prevalent earlier in the sleep period; therefore, sleep terrors typically occur during the first third of the night. REM sleep occurs later in the sleep period making nightmares more common in the early morning hours.

18. Polysomnography (PSG) is routinely indicated for the diagnosis of sleep-related breathing disorders (both obstructive and central sleep apnea) and periodic limb movement disorder. PSG is also commonly performed during CPAP titration, preoperative evaluation before upper airway surgery for snoring, and follow-up after certain treatment modalities.

19. Advantages of portable sleep recordings include accessibility, convenience, patient acceptability, a familiar sleep environment, and cost savings. The main limitation is the lack of a technician, which may lead to inadequate data due to artifacts or lost leads and inability to titrate CPAP, if needed.

20. Actigraphy is not indicated for the routine diagnosis of any sleep disorder but may play a role in the assessment and treatment response for insomnia, circadian rhythm disturbances, sleep state misperception syndrome, and restless leg syndrome/periodic limb movement disorder (RLS/PLMD).

21. An arousal is defined as a 3-second or longer shift in EEG frequency preceded by a minimum of 10 seconds of any stage of sleep; however, an arousal from REM sleep must include 3 seconds or more of EEG shift and a simultaneous increase in chin electromyography activity.

22. An "epoch" of a PSG has traditionally been defined as a 30-second page or screen of data. This is the basic unit or page used for analyzing and reporting PSG data.

23. EEG frequencies encountered during polysomnography include beta (16–25 Hertz), alpha (8–12 Hertz), theta (3–7 Hertz), and delta (< 2 Hertz).

24. A K-complex is a diphasic waveform with a slow, negative (upward) EEG waveform, immediately followed by a positive (downward) component. It is commonly followed by a spindle, or burst of alpha (known as K-alpha).

25. Sleep spindles display a frequency of 12 to16 Hertz. Their shape has been compared to a full or empty spinning-wheel thread spindle, with paired increasing/decreasing or decreasing/increasing amplitudes.

26. Sleep spindles are generated in the reticular nucleus of the thalamus and are thought to "deafferent" or decrease afferent input into the cortex. In other words, spindles decrease external stimulation to the cortex and therefore are thought to facilitate sleep.

27. Between 20-50% of an epoch must be delta sleep to be defined as stage III sleep, but greater than 50% of the epoch must be delta sleep to be defined as stage IV sleep.

28. Saw-tooth waves are seen during REM sleep. Saw-tooth waves have theta frequency and are more prominent in the central leads. They are repetitive with well-delineated positive and negative components of equivalent height or amplitude (like the teeth of a saw).

29. Obstructive apneas occur when the airway closes off with continued respiratory effort; while central apneas occur when respiratory effort ceases leading to absence of airflow.

30. Mixed apneas are present when respiratory effort ceases, the airway collapses, and respiratory efforts begin again against the obstructed airway. Most mixed apneas appear as a central apnea followed by an obstructive apnea.

31. An apnea is defined as decreased nasal-oral airflow to less than 20% compared with baseline and lasting at least 10 seconds. An obstructive apnea requires evidence for continued respiratory effort as measured by abdominal and/or thoracic monitoring.

32. A hypopnea is defined as 20–80% decrement in nasal-oral airflow compared with baseline, accompanied by either a 4% oxyhemoglobin desaturation or an EEG arousal.

33. Studies of snoring report a prevalence rate of 32% in men and a prevalence rate of 21% in women.

34. Sleep apnea-hypopnea syndrome (SAHS) is a newer term synonymous term for obstructive sleep apnea (OSA); obesity hypoventilation syndrome (OHS) is the newer, preferred term for Pickwick or pickwickian syndrome.

35. The prevalence of SAHS is 9% for females and 24% for males if an apnea-hypopnea index (AHI) of 5 or greater is used as the definition. The prevalence, using an AHI of 5 or greater with associated symptoms of SAHS, is 2% for females and 4% for males.

36. In patients evaluated for possible sleep-disordered breathing, the oropharyngeal examination should include an evaluation for a low-lying palate, large tongue, enlarged tonsils, and craniofacial abnormalities.

37. Common presenting symptoms for adult patients with SAHS include snoring, snorting, choking, gasping, witnessed apneas, morning headaches, impotence, nocturia, and daytime sleepiness.

38. Common presenting symptoms for children with SAHS include hyperactivity and poor school performance.

39. Risk factors for SAHS include obesity, male gender, postmenopausal status, craniofacial abnormalities, and abnormal upper airway anatomy (i.e., macroglossia or enlarged tonsils). Environmental factors, including alcohol use, smoking, and use of sedative medication, may produce or worsen SAHS.

40. Patients with sleep apnea mainly in the supine position are labeled as having "positional apnea." Although an exact definition is lacking, generally the diagnosis is made if the majority of respiratory events occur while the patient is supine.

41. The standard treatment for SAHS is continuous positive airway pressure (CPAP). Other treatment options depend on symptoms and severity but may include weight loss, surgical therapy, pharmacologic agents, positional therapy, and oral appliances.

42. Weight loss as a treatment for SAHS can be highly effective, although maintaining weight loss is often difficult.

43. Compliance with CPAP is generally designated as at least 4 hours of usage on a nightly basis, which is typically the amount needed for adequate daytime performance. Long-term compliance can often be predicted by the compliance rate after 1 to 2 weeks of CPAP therapy in the majority of patients.

44. Oral appliances show a success rate, defined as a reduction in the AHI by 50%, of 54–81%, whereas 51–64% have an AHI less than 10. Oral appliances are less likely to be curative with severe SAHS and have shown a higher curative rate in patients with mild-to-moderate positional SAHS.

45. Two large prospective studies of middle-aged and older adults (Sleep Heart Health Study and the Wisconsin Sleep Cohort Study) have established a positive association between SAHS and systemic hypertension.

46. Patients with systolic heart failure have an increased prevalence of SAHS and central sleep apnea.

47. Sinus bradycardia and sinus arrhythmia are the most common arrhythmias reported in normal people during sleep.

48. Insomnia is quite common, with surveys reporting that about one-third of all adults had difficulty sleeping at some point in the prior year. About 10% of all adults report the problem as chronic or severe.

49. There are two nosologic systems for diagnosing types of insomnia: the International Classification of Sleep Disorders (ICSD; American Sleep Disorders Association, 1997) and the Diagnostic and Statistical Manual-IV (DSM-IV; American Psychiatric Association, 1994).

50. There are two main categories of treatment for primary insomnia: cognitive-behavioral therapy and pharmacologic treatment.

51. Cognitive-behavioral therapy (CBT) is an umbrella term that refers to a number of different treatments that employ changes in behavior or cognition to improve sleep. Behavioral treatments used for insomnia include sleep restriction therapy, stimulus control therapy, and progressive muscle relaxation. Cognitive therapy seeks to eliminate irrational beliefs about sleep and fears of not sleeping.

52. Sleep hygiene refers to a set of factors that are required for maintenance of a normal sleep-wake pattern. Common examples include maintenance of a regular sleep-wake schedule, limiting use of caffeine and alcohol, avoiding naps, eliminating noise and light from the sleep environment, and not looking at the clock during the night.

53. Hypersomnolence, sleep paralysis, cataplexy, and hypnagogic or hypnopompic hallucinations are considered the cardinal symptoms or "tetrad" of narcolepsy. Some refer to the "pentad" of narcolepsy, including disrupted nighttime sleep.

54. The likelihood that a patient with narcolepsy will have an affected offspring is 1%, which is much higher than the general population.

55. Laughter is the most common emotion trigger for cataplexy, although other strong emotions such as anger or fear may trigger cataplexy as well.

56. An MSLT following a nocturnal polysomnogram can provide electrophysiologic evidence supporting the diagnosis of narcolepsy. Typical findings include a mean sleep latency of less than 5 minutes and 2 or more SOREMPs (sleep-onset REM periods) during the MSLT.

57. There is no genetic test diagnostic for narcolepsy. HLA typing for DQB1 0602 or DR2 has limited diagnostic value since it is present in 20-35% of the general population.

58. The diagnosis of idiopathic hypersomnolence is made in patients younger than age 25 with sleepiness lasting at least 6 months, after elimination of other causes of excessive daytime sleepiness.

59. Stimulant medications used to treat the symptom of daytime sleepiness in narcolepsy and other forms of hypersomnolence include modafinil, methylphenidate, and dextroamphetamine.

60. Primary restless legs syndrome (RLS) is thought to be due to dysfunction of the dopaminergic system. Supplementing dopamine with levodopa or dopaminergic agonists often improve the symptoms of this disease.

61. Iron supplementation in patients who have RLS and ferritin levels less than 50 mg/dl can improve symptoms.

62. Causes of secondary RLS include renal disease, iron deficiency anemia, pregnancy, peripheral neuropathy, antidepressant medication, and agents blocking dopamine receptors (e.g., antipsychotics and metoclopramide).

63. Periodic limb movement disorder (PLMD) is diagnosed by monitoring the activity of the anterior tibialis muscle of the legs (and arm muscle activity, if appropriate) during polysomnography.

64. When sleep-disordered breathing is treated with CPAP, periodic limb movements may improve, remain unchanged, or become more severe. Most patients that develop periodic limb movements after the initiation of CPAP do not require treatment since this may be a short-term phenomenon without long-term consequences.

65. Neurodegenerative diseases that share the pathologic classification of synucleinopathies, including Lewy body disease, multiple system atrophy and Parkinson's disease, have a high association with REM sleep behavior disorder.

66. REM sleep behavior disorder typically occurs during the last half of the night when the majority of REM sleep occurs.

67. In the feline model of REM sleep behavior disorder, lesions of the peri-locus coeruleus result in dream enactment behavior.

68. REM sleep behavior disorder can be effectively treated with clonazepam in the majority of patients.

69. Sleepwalking, or somnambulism, typically occurs during the first third of the night when the majority of slow-wave sleep occurs.

70. Sleep terrors, or pavor nocturnus, are typically described as beginning with an intense scream or cry with the hallmark signs of increased autonomic activity manifested as tachycardia, tachypnea, diaphoresis, high blood pressure, and increased muscle tone.

71. Coexistent sleep disorders, stressors, poor sleep hygiene, and sleep insufficiency may exacerbate parasomnias.

72. Sleep-related violence can arise out of a partial arousal from either REM or NREM sleep. The attack behavior may be against property, another person, or the self.

73. A factor taken into account when a patient has committed sleep-related violence is a history of parasomnia events, such as nocturnal enuresis past the age of 5 years old.

74. Dreaming is reported 85% of the time when people are awakened during REM sleep.

75. Dream recall varies from person to person and depends on such factors as motivation, depth of sleep, verbal skills, and personality. Generally women report more frequent recall than men.

76. Nightmares differ from dreams in that nightmares are frightening enough to awaken the sleeper.

77. REM sleep is thought to be protective against seizure activity in most cases due to its mixed frequency and lack of synchronization. Slow-wave sleep is thought to promote seizure activity due to its high voltage and synchronization.

78. Secondary palatal myoclonus is one of the few movement disorders that persist during sleep. The tremor associated with Parkinson's disease has been recorded during stage I sleep, and tics have been recorded during sleep as well.

79. Patients with myotonic dystrophy have a greater severity of daytime sleepiness not related to an underlying sleep disorder, but the cause is unknown.

80. Side effects of dopaminergic medications include vivid dreaming, hallucinations, and insomnia.

81. Benzodiazepines shorten sleep latency, reduce arousals and awakenings, and increase total sleep time.

82. The polysomnographic findings associated with benzodiazepine use are excessive spindling seen on the EEG and suppressed slow-wave sleep.

83. Acute alcohol ingestion causes increased slow wave sleep. Once the alcohol is metabolized, REM rebound and fragmentation of sleep occur.

84. Infant sleep is divided into active-REM sleep, quiet sleep, and indeterminate sleep.

85. Limit-setting disorder, which occurs when parents/caregivers inconsistently reinforce bedtime limits, results in stalling or refusing to go to bed at an appropriate time.

86. Sleep-onset association disorder occurs when children are unable to fall asleep without a certain object (e.g., pacifier, bottle) or situation (e.g., nursing, rocking).

87. There is an 80–90% chance that a child with sleep terrors or sleep-walking has an affected first-degree relative.

88. Risk factors for sleep-disordered breathing in children include enlarged tonsils and adenoids, obesity, craniofacial abnormalities, and abnormal upper airway tone associated with neurologic disorders.

89. There are no normative data for an apnea-hypopnea index in children.

90. The "sleep and arousal hypothesis" regarding sudden infant death syndrome (SIDS) says that infants at increased risk of SIDS (at 2 months of age) lose the protective response of arousing in response to hypoxia during sleep.

91. Prone position of infants during sleep is a risk factor for SIDS, which led to the recommendation of the supine position. This recommendation has resulted in a decrease in the incidence of SIDS.

92. Primary enuresis occurs when the child has never had a dry period for more than 3 months. Secondary sleep-related enuresis occurs when enuresis redevelops in a child who was formerly "continuously "dry" for at least 3 months.

93. Enuresis may be treated with pharmacologic agents, behavior modifications, and operant conditioning devices such as noise at the time bedwetting occurs.

94. An increased risk of sleep-disordered breathing is found in infants and children with Pierre-Robin syndrome, Goldenhar's syndrome, trisomy 21, Treacher Collins syndrome and velo-cardiofacial syndrome.

95. The prevalence of SAHS in Down's syndrome is 30–60%. This rate is independent of age, obesity, and presence of congenital heart disease.

96. Core body temperature reaches its nadir (CBTmin) 1.5–2 hours prior to habitual morning arising time; melatonin reaches it maximum just before CBTmin.

97. Phase delays are optimally achieved through phototherapy delivered several hours prior to CBTmin, while phase advances are optimally achieved through phototherapy timed to occur in the window several hours after the CBTmin.

98. Patients with non–24-hr sleep-wake disorder or "hypernychthemeral syndrome" have a progressively delayed bedtime and waketime, whereas patients with irregular sleep-wake pattern do not have a single major nocturnal sleep episode or consolidated daytime wake episode.

99. Exogenous melatonin in the dose range of 1–5 mg taken 30 minutes before going to bed may allow for prolonged daytime sleep in patients with shift work sleep disorder.

100. For all of the circadian rhythm sleep disorders, a sleep/wake diary is an inexpensive, reliable way to estimate sleep/wake patterns over a 1- to 2-week interval. For patients who cannot complete the diary, use of a wrist actigraph is an alternative.

I. Background, Evaluation and Monitoring

1. SLEEP MEDICINE: HISTORY AND LITERATURE

Damien Stevens, MD

1. When was the first scoring manual for sleep recordings published?
Allan Rechtschaffen, MD, and Anthony Kales, MD, published *A Manual of Standardized Terminology, Techniques and Scoring System for Sleep Stages of Human Subjects* while working at UCLA in 1968.

2. What is Yogi Berra's well-known quotation about sleep?
As usual, Mr. Berra does not disappoint. He reportedly said, "If I didn't wake up, I'd still be sleeping."

3. What did Hippocrates write about sleep?
Around 400 BC Hippocrates wrote, "Both sleep and wakefulness, when immoderate, are bad." His statment probably remains true even in the modern era. He also mentioned symptoms of sleep apnea.

4. What did Homer write about sleep?
"Even where sleep is concerned, too much is a bad thing"—quite similar to Hippocrates' writing. In *The Iliad* Homer calls sleep "the brother of death."

5. What did Aristotle write about sleep?
Aristotle wrote, "That all animals partake in sleep is obvious from the following considerations. The animal is defined by the possession of sensation, and we hold that sleep is in some way the immobilization or fettering of sensation, and that the release or relaxation of this is waking."

6. What did Sir William Osler write about sleep?
In 1906 Sir William Osler observed, "An extraordinary phenomenon in excessively fat young persons is an uncontrollable tendency to sleep—like the fat boy in Pickwick." This is one of the first references to Charles Dickens' famous character Joe in his novel, *The Posthumous Papers of the Pickwick Club*. Osler also described many of the presenting signs and symptoms of sleep apnea in the pediatric population and even mentioned the benefit of tonsillectomy in such patients.

7. What did Shakespeare write about sleep?
Shakespeare referred to sleep as "chief nourisher in life's feast" and "balm of minds, great nature's second course." He also wrote, "Not poppy, nor mandragora, nor all the drowsy syrups of the world, shall ever medicine thee to that sweet sleep which thous owedst yesterday." He even described a character, Sir John Falstaff in *Henry IV*, who probably had sleep apnea. Falstaff was overweight, snored loudly, and had daytime hypersomnolence.

8. What did Sigmund Freud write about sleep?
Freud theorized that dreaming functioned as a "safety valve" for the release of instinctual energy. The field of psychoanalysis, which he developed, was based on the interpretation of dreams.

9. Historically, what was the explanation for the physiologic function of sleep?

There are several different theories about the function of sleep. Most theories are based on animal studies since few human data are available. Moruzzi developed a theory that sleep was necessary for recovery and stabilization of synaptic processes. Krueger and colleagues published the theory that nighttime neuronal activity protected neural cells that were not used during the day. Kavanau had a similar idea that sleep allowed "protected" stabilization of these neural cells.

10. When were the first studies of the effects of sleep deprivation?

In the 1920s Kleitman studied the effects of sleep deprivation on daytime impairment. However, Dement published the first major study, entitled "The Depth of Sleep and Dream Deprivation," in 1960. This study first reported the rapid-eye-movement (REM) "pressure" that developed when subjects were deprived of REM sleep.

11. What is the longest time a person has stayed awake?

To date, the record is held by Robert McDonald. He stayed awake for 18 days, 21 hours, and 40 minutes in 1980.

12. Who first described REM sleep?

Eugene Aserinsky, a graduate student of Nathaniel Kleitman at the University of Chicago during the 1920s, published one of the earliest papers about rapid eye movements. Although earlier publications had noted rapid eye movements, they were not analyzed scientifically. Early publications described eye movements first in infants, then later in adults. Initially the subjects' eyes were simply observed, but later authors used electrooculography to electrically record the eye movements. They also recorded dream recall and reported the first association of rapid eye movements with dreaming.

13. What major catastrophes have been attributed, at least in part, to sleep deprivation?

Although the theories are difficult to prove unequivocally, a congressional commission believed that insufficient sleep at least contributed to the nuclear disaster of Chernobyl and the Exxon Valdez accident. Hypersomnolence due to multiple reasons has been hypothesized to lead to innumerable other industrial and personal accidents/injuries.

14. What animal models have been used most commonly to study different areas of sleep medicine?

Rats have commonly been used to study effects of sleep deprivation, and cats are often used to study the neurophysiology of the sleep state, especially REM sleep. Doberman pinschers and Labrador retrievers are the animal models most often used to study narcolepsy. Bulldogs and other breeds have recently been used to study obstructive sleep apnea.

15. Historically, what was the explanation for dream activity?

Early humans seemed to associate dreaming with the "spirit world," but by Plato's time dreams were thought to reflect an unconscious drive. This theory persisted until Freud's psychoanalytic theory.

16. When was obstructive sleep apnea first described?

In 1965, both Gastaut et al. and Jung and Kuhlo first described "Pickwick" syndrome associated with abnormal nocturnal breathing. The first case series was reported in 1978 by Guilleminault and colleagues.

17. When was continuous positive airway pressure (CPAP) first invented?

CPAP was first described in 1981 by Sullivan and colleagues in Australia. They published in *Lancet* their experience using CPAP in 5 patients with severe sleep apnea.

18. What different inventions have been used in the past for the treatment of snoring?
Countless numbers of different devices have been patented or at least submitted for patent for the treatment of snoring. Some of the more entertaining ones are shown in Figures 1–3

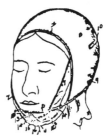

Figure 1. Antisnoring appliance. (From Hoffstein V: Snoring. Chest 109: 201–222, 1996, with permission.)

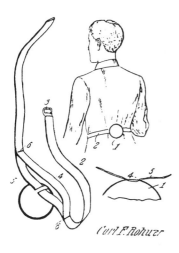

Figure 2. Snore ball. (From Fairbanks DNF: Snoring: A general overview with historical perspective. In Fairbanks DNF, Mickelson SA, Woodson BT (eds): Snoring and Obstructive Sleep Apnea, 3rd ed. Philadelphia, Lippincott Williams & Wilkins, 2003, p 2, with permission).

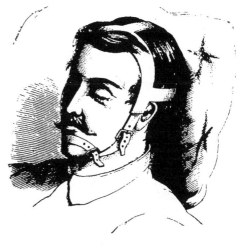

Figure 3. Chin-and-mouth strap. (From Fairbanks DNF: Snoring: A general overview with historical perspective. In Fairbanks DNF, Mickelson SA, Woodson BT (eds): Snoring and Obstructive Sleep Apnea, 3rd ed. Philadelphia, Lippincott Williams & Wilkins, 2003, p 2, with permission.)

19. Who did the first recordings now used in polysomnography?

While at the University of Chicago, Kleitmen first continuously recorded electroencephalograms (EEGs) and eye movements throughout the entire night in the 1950s. However, Hans Berger, a German psychiatrist, described the use of scalp electrodes to record brain activity during both awake and sleep states in 1929.

20. Did "Little Joe" have obstructive sleep apnea?

Most agree that Charles Dickens' character, "Little Joe," probably had severe sleep apnea since he was overweight and excessively sleepy, snored, and was described as "rather slow." However, he may not have been a classic case because he was a child, was noted only to "snore feebly," and also suffered from "dropsy," the historical term for edema. Some believe that his condition may have been related to enlarged tonsils and adenoids rather than a typical case of adult obstructive sleep apnea. Some have also suggested that the character may have had obesity-hypoventilation syndrome in addition to or instead of sleep apnea.

21. When were "restless legs" first described?

Most sleep experts agree the first description was in 1683 by Thomas Willis. Willis described "leapings and contractions of the tendons." The term *restless legs* was first used by K.A. Ekbom in 1945.

22. Who was the Greek god of sleep?

Hypnos, who is also called Sleep in English translations. He was usually described as a sleepy-eyed young man or an older man with a beard. He was a twin of the god of death (Thanatos) and son of the god of night (Nyx). Hypnos had sons known as the gods of dreams, including Morpheus, Icelus, and Phantasus.

23. Who was the Roman god of sleep?

Somnus was the Roman equivalent of Hypnos.

24. How have the average hours of sleep changed over the centuries?

Although reports vary according to age of the population and the years sampled, overall the average sleep length seems to have decreased over the past century. One study of children aged 8 to 17 years found a decrease of 1.5 hours from 1910 to 1963. The accuracy of some of these data has been questioned, however. Another American Cancer Society survey of healthy 50- to 65-year-old subjects found a decrease of 1 hour in the modal sleep hours from 1959 to the 1980s.

25. Who developed the multiple sleep latency test (MLST)?

The MLST was developed by Carskadon and colleagues during studies to measure what determines sleepiness. The earliest publication appeared in 1978.

26. Who developed the maintenance of wakefulness test (MWT)?

The MWT was first reported in 1982 by Mitler and his colleagues. They used this test to evaluate 10 narcoleptic patients. They found that despite patients' claims of alertness, many were unable to stay awake.

27. When was narcolepsy first described?

Jean Baptiste Edouard Gellineau published what most people believe is the first description in 1880.

28. Who first described the genetics of narcolepsy?

Emmanuel Mignot identified a gene linked to narcolepsy in 1999 while working at Stanford University. His research involved dogs but also allowed insight into the human pathophysiology of narcolepsy.

29. Which United States presidents had sleep disorders?

No details are available since polysomnography results have never been reported for any prior president. However, many of the early presidents were noted to be snorers. According to Fairbanks (2003), "Twenty of the thirty-two Presidents of the United States are proved or believed . . . to have been nocturnal nuisances in the White House." William Howard Taft most likely had obstructive sleep apnea due to his obesity. He weighed 350 pounds at his peak weight and was known to snore loudly. Theodore Roosevelt was once noted to snore so loudly that nearly every patient in the hospital wing where he was staying complained.

30. According to the *Guinness Book of World Records*, who is the loudest recorded snorer?

The 1986 edition states that the loudest recorded sound level was 87.5 decibels at Hever Castle in Kent, England in 1984. The snorer was Melvyn Switzer of Hampshire, England. His wife was reportedly deaf in one ear. For a sense of perspective, a jet engine typically produces a sound level of 120 decibels.

31. When was the first book devoted to sleep published?

Edward Binns, MD, published *The Anatomy of Sleep* in 1846. There was very little scientific basis for the text, which consists mostly of anecdotes.

32. Summarize the history of circadian research in sleep medicine.

Jean Jacques d'Ortous deMairan studied circadian rhythms in plants. Some of the earliest studies in humans were performed by Jurgen Aschoff and Rutger Wever of the Max Planck Institute in Germany. They used underground laboratories in their circadian studies.

33. What famous trials have used a "sleep disorder" as a defense for criminal behavior?

Several defendants have used parasomnia as a defense in criminal cases. The charges against these defendants have ranged from indecent exposure to homicide. Such behavior may be due to sleep walking, homicidal somnambulism (in a murder case), or REM behavior disorder. This defense has had mixed success in different courts.

34. Why was being buried during a deep sleep or coma such a concern in the past?

Fears of "premature interment," sometimes warranted, undoubtedly have existed since humankind has performed burials. This fear seems to have peaked in the late 18th century. During this period special horns and other methods were used as "live tests" to wake people thought to be dead and thus prevent the possibility of premature interment.

35. Is African sleeping sickness a sleep disorder?

Sleeping sickness has been endemic in tropical Africa for centuries but was unknown to the rest of the world until European colonies were established in the late 19th century. Albert Schweitzer cared for many patients with this disease during his time in central Africa. The disease is due to a protozoan, the African trypanosome, with the tsetse fly as its vector. The sleep-wake cycle and other biologic rhythms are disrupted. Eventually patients develop dementia and decreased levels of consciousness.

36. What did Native Americans believe about sleep?

Many tribes thought that breathing through the nose was healthier than breathing through the mouth. George Catlin described this observation in a book that was widely published in the 1800s under the title, *The Breath of Life,* and later as *Shut Your Mouth and Save Your Life*. He observed American Indians sleeping peacefully in the supine position and breathing through the nose with their mouth shut. He thought that this sleeping pattern played a role in their vigorous health and warned of the adverse health effects of mouth breathing.

37. What famous gunfighter reportedly shot a man for loud snoring?

John Wesley Hardin supposedly shot a man who was snoring loudly in an adjacent hotel room.

38. What references do religious texts make to sleep and dreaming?

The Bible makes more than 100 references to sleep, many in the book of Psalms. One of the most interesting passages is found in the book of Samuel, which states, "The deepest sleep resembles death." The Koran and the Talmud make fewer references to sleep. Of note, however, the Talmud compares sleep and death: "Sleep and death are similar . . . sleep is one-sixtieth of death."

39. Who was Ondine? What was her curse?

Ondine was a beautiful water nymph from Greek literature, but her story has been told in many different versions and with many cultural variations. Nymphs were immortal unless they fell in love with a mortal and bore a child. The most common version of this legend involves an unfaithful knight named Sir Lawrence and Ondine, a water nymph who fell in love with him. His wedding vow, "My every waking breath shall be my pledge of love and faithfulness to you," eventually backfires when Ondine finds him with another woman years later. She curses him with the promise, "As long as you are awake, you shall have your breath, but should you ever fall asleep, that breath will be taken from you and you will die." Therefore, Ondine's curse is the eponym given for central alveolar hypoventilation, which is usually congenital.

40. Who was Rip Van Winkle?

Washington Irving wrote the story of Rip Van Winkle in 1819-1820, along with "The Legend of Sleepy Hollow," in a collection called *The Sketch Book*. Both stories are actually based on German folklore. Rip Van Winkle fell asleep while in the woods and woke up 20 years later. The setting was the period just after the Revolutionary War, and the story focuses on how time and changes in the world affect life.

41. What is the story behind the legend of Sleeping Beauty?

The legend of Sleeping Beauty seemingly comes from an old Arthurian romance entitled "Perceforest." Folklore probably preceded this version, but the history remains unclear. The story evolved over time with several different versions, but eventually the brothers Grimm recorded a tamer version in the 19th century, the common version in the modern era.

42. What did Lord Byron write regarding sleep?

Sleep hath its own world,
And a wide realm of wild reality,
And dreams in their development have breath,
And tears, and tortures, and the touch of Joy.

BIBLIOGRAPHY

1. Dement WC, Vaughan C (eds): The Promise of Sleep. New York, Random House, 1999.
2. Dement WC: History of sleep physiology and medicine. In Kryger MH, Roth T, Dement WC (eds): Principles and Practice of Sleep Medicine, 3rd ed. Philadelphia, W.B. Saunders, 2000, pp 1–14.
3. Fairbanks DNF: Snoring: A general overview with historical perspective. In Fairbanks DNF, Mickelson SA, Woodson BT (eds): Snoring and Obstructive Sleep Apnea, 3rd ed. Philadelphia, Lippincott Williams & Wilkins, 2003, pp 1–17.
4. Hoffstein V: Snoring. Chest 109:201–222, 1996.

2. HUMAN SLEEP

Aiman Tulaimat, MD, and Babak Mokhlesi, MD

NORMAL SLEEP

1. What are the proposed functions of sleep?

The exact reason why we sleep has not been completely elucidated. The fact that all animals need sleep makes it a necessity of life. Several possible functions of sleep have been proposed:

- Memory consolidation (see question 38).
- Energy conservation: during sleep energy expenditure and oxygen consumption are reduced and the levels of energy substrates such as adenosine triphosphate (ATP) increase in the brain.
- Brain restoration: sleep is the period for brain and body growth, as supported by the increase in growth hormone release during sleep.
- Protective behavioral adaptation: periods of darkness avoid exposure to predators.
- Immune function regulation: experimental data support deterioration of immune function due to sleep deprivation.

2. What are the types and stages of sleep?

Sleep is divided into two main types: non-rapid-eye-movement (NREM) sleep and rapid-eye-movement (REM) sleep. NREM sleep and REM sleep are as different from one another as each is from wakefulness. NREM sleep is divided into four stages based on the electroencephalogram (EEG): stages 1 through 4. The arousal threshold increases from its nadir in stage 1 to its peak in stage 4. The two types of REM sleep are based on the absence or presence of short-lived bursts of eye movement: tonic REM and phasic REM, respectively.

3. How does normal sleep progress in a young adult?

As a young adult falls into the first cycle of sleep, the EEG activity changes pattern from alpha activity (8–13 Hertz or cycles per second [cps]) to a relatively low-voltage mixed frequency pattern (stage 1) that lasts 1–7 minutes. Stage 2 follows stage 1, lasts 10–25 minutes, and is characterized by K-complexes and sleep spindles. Stage 2 progresses into slow-wave sleep (stages 3 and 4) that is characterized by low-frequency (< 2 Hertz), high-voltage activity (75 mV). Stage 3, defined as slow-wave sleep (SWS) activity, accounts for 20–50% of EEG activity, lasts a few minutes, and is followed by stage 4. Stage 4 is defined as SWS, accounts for more than 50% of EEG activity, and typically lasts 20–40 minutes. REM sleep follows stage 1 or 2 of NREM sleep and is short-lived in the first cycle of sleep. REM sleep is characterized by low-voltage, fast EEG, suppression of muscle tone, and rapid eye movements. The duration of REM sleep cycles increases from the first to the last full sleep cycle. The longest REM sleep cycle occurs toward the end of normal sleep and may last as long as an hour. Therefore, the percentage of SWS is highest in the first cycle of sleep, whereas REM sleep is more predominant toward the morning hours. Typical hypnograms of the three major age groups are shown in Figure 1.

4. What is the duration of NREM-REM cycle? How many cycles are there in a night's sleep?

In a night's sleep, four to six full sleep cycles are observed. The average length of the first NREM-REM cycle is 70–100 minutes while the following cycles average 90–120 minutes.

5. What are the characteristics of NREM sleep?

- NREM sleep is characterized by synchronized EEG activity, slow or no eye movements, and tonically active electromyogram (although typically unmoving).

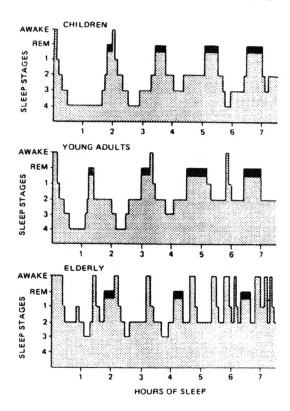

Figure 1. Typical hypnograms from children, young adults, and elderly subjects. (From Chokroverty S: Sleep Disorder Medicine, 2nd ed. Boston, Butterworth-Heinemann, 1999, p 11, with permission.)

- Thermoregulatory response to changes in ambient temperature is intact.
- Respiratory pattern is regular.
- Heart rate and blood pressure are lower than during relaxed wakefulness.
- Activity in the brainstem reticular formations is lower than during wakefulness.
- Cerebral blood flow and cerebral glucose utilization are lower than during wakefulness.
- Unfocused thought with occasional short dreams.

6. What are the characteristics of REM sleep?

- REM sleep is also known as paradoxical sleep because the EEG resembles a waking pattern, but the muscles (except extraocular muscles and the diaphragm) are atonic.
- Thermoregulatory response to ambient temperature is absent.
- Tidal volume and breathing frequency are more variable than in NREM sleep.
- Ventilatory response to hypercarbia and hypoxia is reduced in comparison to NREM sleep and wakefulness.
- Heart rate and blood pressure are variable and similar to relaxed wakefulness.
- Cerebral blood flow, glucose utilization, and oxygen consumption are similar to wakefulness.
- Penile erections occur in men.
- Abundant long dreaming with clear recollection of its content.

7. What is an arousal?

The American Academy of Sleep Medicine defines an arousal as a 3-second or longer shift in EEG frequency, including theta, alpha, or > 16 Hertz activity (excluding spindles), preceded by a minimum of 10 seconds of any stage of sleep. Artifacts, K complexes, and delta sleep are not considered arousal unless they occur during the 3 seconds of EEG shift. Since bursts of alpha activity may occur during normal REM sleep, arousal from REM sleep must include 3 seconds or more of EEG shift and a simultaneous increase in electromyography (EMG) activity. Arousal scoring is independent of Rechtschaffen and Kales epoch scoring. Agreement on 3 seconds is methodologic, not physiologic. EEG shifts lasting less than 3 seconds increase interobserver and intraobserver variability.

8. What is considered a normal "arousal index"?

The normal number of arousals per hour of sleep (arousal index), as documented by laboratory polysomnography, is 13 ± 2/hour in teenagers (10–19 years), 14 ± 2/hour in young adults (20–39 years), 18 ± 2/hour in middle-aged adults (40–59), and 27 ± 3/hour in normal elderly subjects (60 years and older). Of interest, the Sleep Heart Health Study investigators reported a similar arousal index (15/hour) during home polysomnography in 1691 middle-aged subjects without sleep-disordered breathing.

9. What are the characteristics of normal sleep in children?

Neonates (38–42 weeks of gestation) sleep about 16 hours per day, equally distributed between night and day. Nighttime sleep gradually consolidates into one uninterrupted block in 90% of infants by the end of the first year, and daytime sleep gradually decreases over the first 3 years. By the age of 4 years, most children do not require a daytime nap.

Before the age of 6 months, infants spend 50% of sleep time in REM sleep. Infants may enter sleep through an initial REM stage. Active REM sleep emerges more often during sleep cycle in infants, resulting in a shorter sleep cycling between NREM and REM (50–60 minutes). After 6 months, the infant's sleep architecture closely resembles that of an adult, and sleep-onset REM sleep disappears. The amplitude of SWS can be as high as 150 mV.

10. Describe the effect of aging on sleep architecture.

The sleep period (time from sleep onset at night until awakening in the morning) does not change with age. In contrast, total sleep time (sleep period minus the duration of awakenings) decreases with age after adulthood, particularly after midlife. The elderly are sleepier and nap more frequently during the day than younger adults. Therefore, the 24-hour sleep amount of elders is probably not different from that of young adults. These changes are probably due to a higher incidence of sleep disorders and age-related changes in the circadian rhythm.

The most common changes in sleep architecture related to aging are a reduction in duration and voltage of SWS, an increase in the number and duration of nocturnal arousals and awakenings, and a slight reduction in REM sleep. The effects of aging on REM sleep are variable and occur later in life. The decrease in SWS occurs in early to mid adulthood. These changes are more prominent in men than in women. In men, the percentage of SWS decreases by 80% from early adulthood to midlife (age 16–25 to 36–50 years). Light sleep (i.e., stages 1 and 2) compensates for this decrease in deep sleep without significant change in wake time. REM sleep does not change from early adulthood to midlife. Beyond midlife, wake time increases, whereas light and REM sleep decrease.

11. What sleep changes accompany pregnancy?

Pregnant women report that during the first trimester total sleep time, daytime sleepiness, and nocturnal awakenings increase, whereas overall sleep quality decreases. Sleep appears to normalize in the second trimester. In the third trimester, women awaken 3–5 times per night, nap an hour during the day, and complain of insomnia and daytime sleepiness. Sleep studies in pregnant women confirming these reports and show that total sleep time increases in the first trimester, normalizes in the second trimester, and decreases in the third trimester. Moreover, slow-wave sleep is reduced throughout pregnancy, and REM sleep is reduced in the third trimester.

12. What sleep changes accompany menopause?

Menopause is associated with poor sleep quality that might be related to either nocturia or the vasomotor symptoms associated with menopause. Hormone replacement therapy subjectively improves sleep initiation and quality. Menopause is also associated with increased prevalence of sleepapnea-hypopnea syndrome (SAHS). The prevalence of SAHS (apnea–hypopnea index >15) in postmenopausal women is 11–12%. Postmenopausal women are more likely than pre-menopausal women to have obstructive sleep apnea (odds ratio: 2.5). The prevalence of SAHS is 40–50% less in postmenopausal women receiving hormone replacement therapy than in women without such replacement.

DETERMINANTS OF SLEEP

13. Explain the "two-process model" for the sleep-wake cycle.

The two-process model is an influential theory proposed by Alexander Borbely. It suggests that sleep-wake propensity results from a combination of an intrinsic circadian pacemaker (process C) and a homeostatic process (process S), as shown in Figure 2. Circadian input cause a greater or lesser tendency for sleep at specific times of the day and provides temporal organization of the sleep-wakefulness cycles. Two circadian peaks for sleep propensity occur per day: in the early morning hours (3–5 AM) and in the early afternoon (2–3 PM). Homeostatic sleep drive increases with increasing time spent awake; the longer the period awake, the greater the propensity to sleep. A third regulator has been proposed, the ultradian REM-NREM oscillator, that should come into play during sleep.

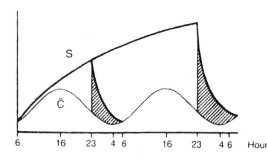

Figure 2. The two-process model involves a sleep homeostatic process (S) and a circadian process (C). Sleep deprivation causes a progressive increase in process S, while fluctuations in process C persist. (From Chokroverty S: Sleep Disorder Medicine, 2nd ed. Boston, Butterworth-Heinemann, 1999, p 143, with permission.)

CIRCADIAN EFFECTS

14. What does the term *circadian* mean?

Circadian activities (from Latin: *circa* = about, *dies* = day) are rhythms with periods approximating 24 hours.

15. What does the term *ultradian* mean?

Ultradian processes are those that repeat with a period of less than 24 hours. For example, the ultradian NREM-REM sleep has a period of 60 minutes in infants and 90–120 minutes in adults.

16. What does the term *infradian* mean?

Infradian processes are multiday rhythms, such as the menstrual cycle.

17. What are the properties of circadian rhythms?
- Circadian rhythms persist without environmental cues.
- All eukaryotic cells have circadian rhythms with periods (τ) that are determined genetically and that are different among species.
- Circadian rhythms are innate and not learned.
- Circadian rhythms are temperature-compensated: the length of the period is invariant over a wide range of temperatures, because whether it is a cold day or a warm day, it is still a 24-hour day.

- Circadian rhythms can be synchronized, or entrained, by external time cues, most notably the daily light-dark cycle.

18. What are *Zeitgebers*?

Zeitgebers (from German: *Ziet* = time, *Geber* = giver) are environmental variables that are capable of entraining circadian rhythm. The most potent zeitgeber is exposure to bright daylight. Nevertheless, lower photic sensitivity on the order of ordinary indoor room lighting also functions as a zeitgeber. Weaker zeitgebers include exercise, social stimuli, temperature, and feeding. Generally, humans do not entrain to zeitgebers with periods greater than 32 hours or less than 18 hours.

19. What is entrainment?

Circadian rhythms are generated by biologic clocks with duration slightly longer than 24 hours. However, they become synchronized to the 24-hour day by environmental stimuli or zeitgebers. Entrainment is the process by which an external process (light-dark cycle) synchronizes the internal pacemaker of an organism. In most humans, entrainment occurs every day when a stimulus (e.g., exposure to light) resets the internal pacemaker to compensate for the difference between the intrinsic period of the pacemaker and the environmental cycle.

20. Define the amplitude and phase of a rhythm.

Amplitude is the magnitude or peak-to-trough difference in a rhythm. **Phase** is a particular point in the cycle.

21. What do the terms *acrophase* and *nadir* mean?

Acrophase is the maximum amplitude of a rhythm. **Nadir** is the minimum amplitude of a rhythm.

22. What does the term *tau* mean?

Tau (τ) is the "endogenous" period of a rhythm. All animal species studied to date and even microorganisms have persistence of daily rhythms in constant conditions generated by an internal, self-sustaining biologic clock. The period (τ) of a free-running rest-activity cycle under constant conditions varies among species and ranges from 23 to 26 hours.

23. What is a tau mutation?

It is a mutation in the golden hamster that arose spontaneously in laboratory stock. Cultures of retinal cells from wild-type golden hamster exhibit a circadian rhythm of melatonin production with a 24-hour period. Tau mutation reduces the circadian period from 24 hours to 22 hours in heterozygote hamsters and to 20 hours in homozygote hamsters.

24. What is meant by the term *forced desynchrony*? How is it useful?

Forced desynchronization is a method used to overcome the difficulty in studying the contribution of process C and S to sleep. During a forced desynchronization protocol, a light-dark cycle with a 28-hour period is imposed on the studied subject, who has a normal 24.2-hour internal clock period. This situation leads to desynchronization of circadian and homeostatic factors and permits the study of sleep and wakefulness at different circadian phases. Such experiments have shown that slow-wave activity is driven mainly by homeostatic factors, whereas spindle activity and REM sleep are driven by circadian factors.

HOMEOSTATIC EFFECTS AND SLEEP DEPRIVATION

25. How is sleep homeostatically conserved?

In humans and animals, the depth of sleep is proportional to the duration of wakefulness preceding it. Deep sleep or SWS is characterized by an increase in arousal threshold. This increase in arousal threshold renders the individual difficult to arouse and ensures a restorative continuous sleep.

26. What is the neurobiologic substrate underlying sleep homeostasis (somnogenes)?

Adenosine may be the basis of the homeostatic sleep need. In the central nervous system, an increase in neuronal activity enhances energy consumption as well as extracellular adenosine concentrations. In most brain areas, high extracellular adenosine concentrations, through A1 adenosine receptors, decrease neuronal activity and thus the need for energy. Adenosine seems to act as a direct negative feedback inhibitor of neuronal activity. It is hypothesized that during prolonged wakefulness accumulating adenosine inhibits specific anterior hypothalamic and basal forebrain neurons containing gamma-aminobutyric acid; this process, in turn, inhibits the sleep-active ventrolateral preoptic nucleus neurons. Disinhibited sleep-active gamma-aminobutyric acid neurons of the ventrolateral preoptic nucleus and adjacent structures inhibit the wake-active histaminergic, aminergic, and cholinergic ascending arousal systems, thereby initiating NREM sleep.

27. How much sleep do humans need?

There is large variability in the need for sleep. Most people sleep an average of about 7–8 hours/night. Sleep need may have a normal Gaussian distribution, and individuals may have their own sleep needs. Sleep researchers disagree on the amount of sleep that a normal person needs. Some investigators have introduced the concept of core sleep, defined as the amount of uninterrupted, good-quality sleep (6 hours/night) necessary to repair the effects of waking wear and tear on the brain in order to maintain adequate daytime functioning.

28. How many hours of sleep do most people currently obtain?

Over the past century there has been a gradual decline in the total sleep time in the U.S. population. The 2003 poll on Sleep in America, performed by the National Sleep Foundation, reported that U.S. adults between 18 and 54 years of age sleep on average 6.7 hours during the workweek. Most young adults compensate for sleep loss by sleeping longer on the weekend, with an average increase to 7.6 hours. Only 30% of young adults stated that they get at least 7–8 hours of sleep per night during the workweek; and 40% of adults reported getting fewer than 7 hours of sleep per night during the workweek. The average amount of sleep during the workweek increases with age. In contrast to the elderly, who sleep the same number of hours on weekdays and weekends, young adults sleep an hour longer on the weekends compared with the workweek.

In a controversial observational study, the mortality rate of adults who slept 7 hours per night was lower than that of participants who reported sleeping 8 hours or more and those who slept 6 hours or less. The highest risk was observed in participants reporting more than 8.5 hours or less than 4.5 hours of sleep per day.

29. Define natural short and natural long sleepers.

Natural short (5 hours/night) and long sleepers (10 hours/night) are people who sleep far more or less than the average. The International Classification of Sleep Disorders categorizes both conditions as proposed sleep disorders. Whether these conditions are truly sleep disorders remains controversial. However, they are an important part of the differential diagnoses of people with inability to sleep or excessive sleepiness. Such people may represent the two ends of the presumably normal distribution of sleep need.

30. What are the characteristics of natural short sleepers?

During a 24-hour period, a natural short sleeper sleeps substantially less than expected for a person of the same age. Short sleepers are neither subjectively nor objectively somnolent during the daytime and are unable to sleep longer despite opportunities and attempts to do so. Their sleep is restorative and high-quality. In contrast to people with insufficient sleep, short sleepers do not compensate on weekends for lost sleep. It remains to be elucidated whether short sleepers have a lower need for sleep or higher tolerance to sleep pressure compared with normal individuals.

31. What are the characteristics of natural long sleepers?

During a 24-hour period, a natural long sleeper sleeps substantially more than expected for a person of the same age. The sleep efficiency, timing, and quality are normal. Social demands that reduce the duration of sleep can lead to symptoms of insufficient sleep. Longer sleepers tend to have longer sleep latency and lower sleep efficiency than short sleepers. The absolute amount of SWS is normal, whereasthe absolute amounts of stage 2 and REM sleep are somewhat higher than normal. Long sleepers have no sleep pathology. If consistently allowed to sleep their perceived sleep need, they will not develop daytime sleepiness.

32. How long can a human stay awake?

In 1965, Randy Gardner, a 17-year-old high school student, set the world record by staying awake for 264 hours and 12 minutes. Recovery sleep in the first night was 14.4 hours. In 1980, however, Robert McDonald stayed awake for almost 19 days, surpassing the previous record by several days. In carefully monitored experiments, normal research subjects have remained awake for 8–10 days. None of these subjects experienced serious medical, neurologic, physiologic, or psychiatric problems. However, they showed progressive deficits in concentration, motivation, perception, and other higher mental processes as the duration of sleep deprivation increased. The subjects recovered to relative normality within one or two nights of recovery sleep. Recovery sleep after total sleep deprivation shows an increase in the percentage of SWS. REM sleep percentage may also increase if sleep deprivation is prolonged (> 4 days).

33. What are the effects of sleep deprivation in animals?

Rats die after 3 weeks of total sleep deprivation or after 5 weeks of REM sleep deprivation. Despite a large increase in food intake, sleep-deprived rats lose weight due a doubling of energy expenditure in the face of a drop of body temperature and develop multiple organ failure.

34. What are the behavioral effects of total sleep deprivation in humans?

Tasks most affected by sleep loss are long, monotonous, without feedback, and externally paced (e.g., driving). Sleep-deprived medical residents and patients with sleep apnea have more car accidents than controls in most studies.

35. What are the effects of partial acute sleep deprivation?

Vigilance declines after reducing sleep to 3 hours for one night or to 5 hours for two consecutive nights. All sleep stages are reduced except SWS. If recovery sleep is restricted to 8 hours, total sleep time will be slightly increased with a corresponding decrease in sleep latency. If sleep is allowed ad lib, the increased sleep time consists mostly of stage 2 and REM sleep.

36. What are the effects of partial chronic sleep deprivation?

Chronic restriction of sleep to 4–6 hours per night for 14 consecutive days results in a cumulative dose-dependent deficit in cognitive performance. This finding is in contrast to the increase in subjective sleepiness, which is dose-independent and noncumulative. Chronic restriction of sleep to 6 hours or less leads to deficits in cognitive performance similar to those resulting from two nights of total sleep deprivation. The EEG in chronic sleep deprivation shows a reduction in all sleep stages except SWS with a tendency for an increase in stage 4 sleep. The first recovery night may show a rebound in SWS.

37. What is "microsleep"?

Microsleep is a transient physiologic sleep (3–14 seconds of EEG pattern change from wakefulness to stage 1) with or without rolling eye movements or behavioral sleep (drooping or slight sagging and nodding of the head). The performance decrement that results from sleep deprivation may be due to microsleep.

SLEEP AND MEMORY

38. What is the role of sleep in learning?

Sleep processes participate in the consolidation of memory—the processing of memory traces during which they are reactivated, analyzed, and gradually incorporated into long-term memory. REM sleep, in particular, seems to play a role in the consolidation of procedural learning but not of declarative memory. On the other hand, SWS might be important in the consolidation of declarative memory tasks. The following points clarify these positions:

1. Posttraining sleep deprivation impairs subsequent performance on various tasks. This impairment occurs only if the task entails a new behavior or if sleep deprivation occurred during the so-called "paradoxical sleep windows." Sleep deprivation outside these windows has no effect on subsequent performance.
2. In humans and animals the duration of REM sleep increases after training in various tasks. The duration of REM sleep normalizes once the task is mastered.
3. Brain cell activity of rats as they train to run around a track match the brain activity during sleep. The brain cell activity in zebra finches indicates that during sleep the birds replay songs in their heads, possibly to help secure the memory.
4. Several brain areas activated during various tasks were significantly more active during REM sleep in trained subjects than in nontrained subjects.
5. Sleep is important for procedural memory. In one study, participants had to repeatedly type a sequence on a keyboard. A group trained in the morning and then tested 12 hours later showed no significant improvement. However, a full night's sleep improved their performance by almost 20%. Another group, trained in the evening, improved their performance by about 20% after a full night's sleep.
6. A nap in the middle of the day may benefit some learning processes. Scores on a task that tests procedural memory worsened over the course of four daily practice sessions. This "burnout" occurred because the brain could only take in so much information before it had a chance to secure the memory of it through sleep. A half-hour nap after the second session prevented further deterioration. An hour nap improved performance in sessions done later in the day.

BIBLIOGRAPHY

1. Borbely AA, Tobler I: Endogenous sleep-promoting substances and sleep regulation. Physiol Rev 69:605–670, 1989.
2. Ferrara M, De Gennaro L: How much sleep do we need? Sleep Med Rev 5:155–179, 2001.
3. Kripke DF, Garfinkel L, Wingard DL, et al: Mortality associated with sleep duration and insomnia. Arch Gen Psychiatry 59:131–136, 2002.
4. Mednick SC, Nakayama K, Cantero JL, et al: The restorative effect of naps on perceptual deterioration. Nat Neurosci 5:677–681, 2002.
5. Rechtschaffen A: Current perspectives on the function of sleep. Perspect Biol Med 41:359–390, 1998.
6. Santiago JR, Nolledo MS, Kinzler W, et al: Sleep and sleep disorders in pregnancy. Ann Intern Med 134:396–408, 2001.
7. Sejnowski TJ, Destexhe A: Why do we sleep? Brain Res 886:208–223, 2000.
8. Siegel JM: Mechanisms of sleep control. J Clin Neurophysiol 7:49–65, 1990.
9. Siegel JM: The REM sleep-memory consolidation hypothesis. Science 294:1058–1063, 2001.
10. Van Cauter E, Leproult R, Plat L: Age-related changes in slow wave sleep and REM sleep and relationship with growth hormone and cortisol levels in healthy men. JAMA 284:861–868, 2000.
11. Van Dongen HP, Maislin G, Mullington JM, et al: The cumulative cost of additional wakefulness: Dose-response effects on neurobehavioral functions and sleep physiology from chronic sleep restriction and total sleep deprivation. Sleep 26:117–126, 2003.
12. White DP: The hormone replacement dilemma for the pulmonologist. Am J Respir Crit Care Med 167:1165–1166, 2003.

3. PHYSIOLOGIC CHANGES IN SLEEP

Damien Stevens, MD

NERVOUS SYSTEM

1. What happens to pupillary diameter during sleep?

Pupillary constriction occurs during non-rapid-eye-movement (NREM) sleep because of parasympathetic innervation. This constriction also persists during REM sleep due to the same innervation. However, during phasic REM papillary dilation is due to inhibition of parasympathetic outflow.

2. How is sympathetic activity assessed during sleep?

Sympathetic activity can be assessed by several methods. Catecholamine levels in serum and urine can be measured during sleep. Measures of heart rate variability can also be assessed as indicators of sympathetic activity, but which markers reflect sympathetic activity is not entirely agreed upon. One of the best methods is probably direct measurement of muscle sympathetic nervous activity with microneurography. A small-caliber tungsten microelectrode is placed directly into the muscle, often the peroneal, and direct neural activity can be recorded from the muscle and blood vessel. This recording can then displayed and analyzed (Fig. 1).

3. What happens to parasympathetic and sympathetic tone during NREM sleep?

As a rule, whole body parasympathetic tone is increased and sympathetic tone is decreased during NREM sleep. During arousals, sympathetic tone usually increases in bursts of activity. These bursts of activity may also be associated with K complexes seen during stage 2 sleep.

4. What happens to parasympathetic and sympathetic tone during REM sleep?

During REM sleep, parasympathetic tone is increased even further, whereas sympathetic tone reaches it lowest level. However, during phasic REM periods, sympathetic activity transiently increases, as shown in Figure 1.

5. How does sympathetic tone differ in skeletal muscle compared with splanchnic and renal vessels?

Muscle sympathetic tone is reduced, as noted above, during NREM sleep but during REM sleep muscle sympathetic tone increases to levels above waking values. This increase leads to vasoconstriction in skeletal muscle vessels. In contrast, splanchnic and renal blood vessels vasodilate due to the decreased sympathetic drive to the kidneys and visceral organs during REM sleep.

6. How does limb muscle tone vary in NREM and REM sleep?

Muscle tone is maximal during wakefulness but decreases during NREM sleep and decreases even further or is completely absent during REM sleep. During REM sleep myotonic bursts of different muscle groups can be seen as well "phasic twitches," which are brief, intermittent surges of electromyographic (EMG) activity.

7. How does upper airway muscle tone change in sleep?

There is an overall reduction in activity of the upper airway dilator muscles during NREM sleep; the reduction is even greater during REM sleep. This decreased activity leads to upper airway narrowing and therefore increased upper airway resistance. The main upper airway muscles involved in this process include the genioglossus, palatoglossus, tensor veli palatini, levator veli palatini, and hyoid muscles. During REM sleep muscle atonia exacerbates this process even further.

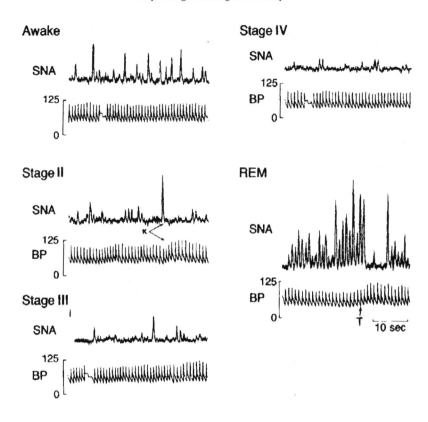

Figure 1. Sympathetic nerve activity (SNA) and blood pressure recordings during awake and different sleep stages. Note the decline in SNA during stages I, II, and IV compared with the awake state as well as the sharp increase during REM sleep. (From Somers VK, Dyken MD, Mark AL, Abboud FM: Sympathetic nerve activity during sleep in normal subjects. N Engl J Med 328:303. 1993, with permission.)

Of interest, upper airway anesthesia in healthy people produces some apneas, probably due to lost reflex activity, but this effect does not occur in patients with sleep apnea-hypopnea syndrome.

RESPIRATORY PHYSIOLOGY

8. What happens to arterial partial pressure of carbon dioxide (pCO_2) during different stages of sleep?
    Arterial pCO_2 typically increases by 2–8 mmHg acutely upon sleep onset.

9. What happens to arterial partial pressure of oxygen (pO_2) during sleep?
    Arterial pO_2 decreases by 3–10 mmHg, and oxygen saturation typically decreases by less than 2% during sleep.

10. How do oxygen consumption and carbon dioxide production change during sleep?
    Oxygen consumption and carbon dioxide production decrease during sleep. This finding is not surprising because muscle activity and sympathetic activity are also decreased during sleep, both leading to a slowing of metabolism.

11. How do tidal volume, respiratory rate, and minute ventilation change during different sleep stages?

Minute ventilation falls by 0.5–1.5 liters per minute during NREM sleep. This decrease is due to a reduction in tidal volume rather than in respiratory rate. During REM sleep the fall in minute ventilation is similar, but this change varies among different studies. Most studies do show a consistent fall of minute ventilation during phasic REM. Respiration also becomes very irregular during phasic REM.

12. How do hypoxic and hypercapnic ventilatory responses change during NREM and REM sleep?

The hypoxic ventilatory response typically decreases during NREM sleep and decreases further during REM sleep. This decrease is thought to be due to decreased chemosensitivity. The hypercapnic ventilatory response decreases in a similar pattern, with a fall during NREM and an additional fall during REM sleep. An increase in upper airway resistance may also play a role in the decreased response to hypoxia and hypercapnia.

13. What typically happens to functional residual capacity during sleep?

Functional residual capacity (FRC) usually declines by 10% during sleep or when people assume the supine position. This fall may be exaggerated in patients with neuromuscular disease or obesity. Typically, a larger reduction in FRC causes a greater decrease in oxygen stores and more severe desaturations.

14. What happens to the cough reflex during sleep?

Cough is normally caused by stimulation of laryngeal receptors. The reflex is attenuated during NREM and REM sleep. This decrease in the cough reflex probably plays a role in the common phenomenon of asymptomatic nocturnal aspiration, which is seen in healthy adults. In infants, stimulation of the larynx may induce apnea episodes. This reflex may play a role in sudden infant death syndrome.

15. Which is a stronger stimulus for arousal—hypercapnia or hypoxemia?

The arousal response to carbon dioxide varies among different studies. Some report no differences related to sleep states, whereas others have shown an increase in arousal responses. Hypoxemia alone is usually a poor stimulus for arousal; severe desaturations are often recorded without arousals. The combination of hypoxemia and hypercapnia appears to be the strongest stimulus for arousal.

CARDIOVASCULAR PHYSIOLOGY

16. What happens to heart rate and cardiac output during sleep?

Heart rate decreases during NREM sleep but fluctuates greatly during REM sleep. The decrease in heart rate seems to be due to increased parasympathetic activity through an increase in vagal activity. The bradytachycardia seen during REM sleep is due to variations of both parasympathetic and sympathetic activity.

Cardiac output falls during both NREM and REM sleep progressively throughout the night. Some believe this fall in cardiac output may play a role in the phenomenon of early morning cardiac ischemia.

17. What is meant by the term *bradytachycardia*?

This term describes the variable episodes of bradycardia and tachycardia, which probably are due to erratic autonomic nervous system activity.

18. What normally happens to pulmonary arterial blood pressure during sleep?

As opposed to systemic blood pressure, pulmonary arterial blood pressure rises, but only slightly, during sleep.

19. What normally happens to systemic arterial blood pressure during sleep?

Like many other cardiac parameters, systemic arterial blood pressure decreases during sleep. During NREM sleep it falls by approximately 10%. During REM sleep, however, blood pressure fluctuates significantly, probably due to sympathetic activity.

20. How do cerebral blood flow and metabolism typically change during sleep?

Cerebral blood flow usually falls by 5–23% during NREM sleep. During REM sleep an increase in blood flow is typically seen, sometimes up to 41% above baseline. Some authors simplify this finding by suggesting that NREM sleep is the "resting" or "inactive" state, whereas REM sleep is a highly "active" neurologic state. However, there is great regional variability in the pattern of increased cerebral blood flow during REM sleep.

21. How does blood flow in the different vascular beds change during sleep?

Blood flow to cutaneous, muscular, and mesenteric beds changes minimally during NREM sleep. During REM sleep blood flow is increased in the mesenteric and renal vascular beds, but vasoconstriction occurs in muscular and cutaneous vessels.

ENDOCRINE PHYSIOLOGY

22. What does deconvolution of hormone levels mean?

This procedure uses a mathematical model that takes into account hormonal distribution and degradation. Hormone secretory rates can then be calculated based on peripheral blood concentrations. Deconvolution allows a more accurate assessment of hormone secretion and its relation to other sleep phenomena.

23. How do different hormones change during sleep?

Figure 2 shows typical changes of some common hormone levels during sleep. It should be remembered that sleep itself may not induce such changes; they may merely coincide with sleep.

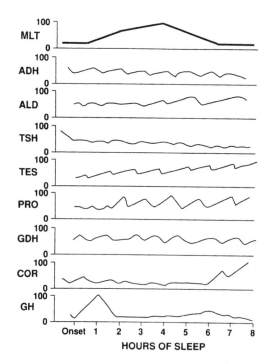

Figure 2. Representative curves of hormone concentrations during sleep. MLT = melatonin, ADH = antidiuretic hormone, ALD = aldosterone, TSH = thyroid-stimulating hormone, TES = testosterone, PRO = prolactin, GDH = gonadotropic hormone, COR= cortisol, GH = growth hormone. (From Chokroverty S: Sleep Disorders Medicine, 2nd ed. Boston, Butterworth-Heinemann, 1999, p 114, with permission.)

Several studies have shown that similar curves may occur in some hormones even during sleep restriction, thereby negating the effect of sleep. As a broad categorization, hormones may be strongly influenced by sleep, minimally influenced by sleep, or influenced by a certain stage of sleep. Prolactin is one of the hormones most strongly influenced by sleep, with a nearly flat curve after sleep restriction. Cortisol secretion, on the other hand, shows minimal influence, with essentially the same secretion pattern even with sleep deprivation. Growth hormone shows pulsatile secretions during slow-wave sleep that are suppressed during sleep restriction.

24. What is the effect of sleep on prolactin?

In general, sleep onset usually stimulates prolactin secretion. In healthy patients with a normal sleep-wake cycle, daytime prolactin levels are relatively low, whereas during the night prolactin levels are increased. An association with specific sleep stages or EEG activity has not consistently been shown in different studies.

25. What is the effect of sleep on gonadotropin hormone (GDH), luteinizing hormone (LH), and follicle-stimulating hormone (FSH)?

GDH is released by the anterior hypothalamus and stimulates the pituitary gland to release LH and FSH. No clear and consistent relationship has been found between any of these hormone levels and sleep.

26. How does sleep affect testosterone levels?

Most studies have shown a consistent rise in testosterone levels during sleep.

27. What is the effect of sleep on thyroid-stimulating hormone (TSH)?

The main effect of sleep appears to be inhibition of TSH secretion. This effect is assumed for several reasons. TSH levels progressively rise throughout the day, with a peak level around the time of sleep onset. During sleep TSH slowly declines through the night.

28. How does sleep affect cortisol?

Cortisol secretion is mainly under endogenous circadian control. As mentioned previously, cortisol levels during normal sleep and sleep restriction show similar curves; thus, it appears that cortisol secretion is independent of sleep. However, some studies have shown a temporal relationship between sleep and cortisol levels. Typically the peak in cortisol levels occurs in the early morning hours.

29. With which stage of sleep is growth hormone (GH) most closely associated?

GH is most closely associated with slow-wave sleep and typically peaks approximately 90 minutes after sleep onset. GH secretion is a marker of slow-wave sleep onset, and a significant correlation has been found between total minutes of slow-wave sleep and GH secretion. The physiologic explanation for this connection remains unknown.

30. What is the affect of sleep on melatonin?

The length of secretion is proportional to the length of sleep, and melatonin release peaks during sleep.

GASTROINTESTINAL PHYSIOLOGY

31. What is the function of the lower esophageal sphincter (LES) during sleep?

The LES is a ringlike band of muscle fibers between the stomach and esophagus; it produces a high pressure that constricts the gastroesophageal junction. The LES has been thought to be the main barrier to gastoesophageal reflux during the day and at night. However, recent studies have shown that patients with normal LES tone still may develop gastroesophageal reflux disease (GERD) and esophageal erosions. Transient relaxations of the LES are thought to lead to GERD, even though a normal baseline tone may be present. LES tone exhibits no circadian variation.

32. Describe the interaction of GERD and sleep.

One study recorded LES tone, esophageal pH, and EEG readings in several patients with GERD and normal controls. The investigators found that most esophageal reflux events were associated with transient relaxation of the LES during awakenings from sleep rather than during sleep. The few events during sleep were usually during stage 2 sleep. The mechanism of this activity is unknown but may be related to episodic increased vagal activity, which causes a decrease in LES tone.

33. What happens to gastric acid production during sleep?

A clear circadian pattern has been shown in healthy patients and patients with ulcers. Basal gastric acid output is greatest in the late evening and lowest in the morning hours. This circadian pattern is not suppressed by H_2 blockers or proton pump inhibitors, but it is abolished by vagotomy.

34. How does sleep affect the function of swallowing?

Swallowing frequency is significantly reduced during sleep. Humans swallow approximately 25 times per hour during the daytime but only 5 times per hour during sleep. Most nocturnal swallowing occurs during movement arousals while the person is in NREM sleep.

35. What happens to gastric and intestinal motility during sleep?

Gastric motility, as measured by gastric slow-wave changes, fluctuates during sleep, with a decrease compared with daytime activity during NREM sleep and a return to normal during REM sleep. There is a delay in gastric emptying during sleep, but esophageal motility shows little circadian variation.

BIBLIOGRAPHY

1. Chokroverty S: Sleep Disorders Medicine, 2nd ed. Boston, Butterworth-Heinemann, 1999.
2. Gronfier C, Brandenberger G: Ultradian rhythms in pituitary and adrenal hormones: Their relations to sleep. Sleep Med Rev 2:17–29, 1998.
3. Lee-Chiong TL, Sateia M, Carskadon MA: Sleep Medicine. Philadelphia, Hanley & Belfus, 2002.
4. Orr WC: Gastrointestinal functioning during sleep: A new horizon in sleep medicine. Sleep Med Rev 5:91–101, 2001.
5. Pasricha PJ: Effect of sleep on gastroesophageal physiology and airway protective mechanisms. Am J Med 115:114S–118S, 2003.

4. NEUROANATOMY AND NEUROPHYSIOLOGY

Suzanne Stevens, MD

1. Is there a "sleep center" in the brain?

The anterior hypothalamus and preoptic areas are thought to be integral to generating sleep. This association was initially noted during the early 1900s when patients with encephalitis lethargica and insomnia were found to have lesions of the anterior hypothalamus. Later experiments in animals showed that stimulation of the anterior hypothalamus and preoptic areas caused behavioral change consistent with sleep. However, this is only one compoent of a complex neuroanatomic pathway, coursing from the brainstem to the cortex, that is thought to be responsible for generating sleep.

2. What makes up the brainstem reticular formation? What is its function?

As shown in Figure 1, the ascending reticular activating system in the brainstem projects via the posterior hypothalamus and subsequently through thalamocortical pathways to the forebrain. This system is necessary to maintain the cortex in an activated state as well as to maintain behavioral wakefulness. This function has been demonstrated experimentally in cats by the *cerveau isolé* procedure, which separates the cortex from the brainstem and results in cortical brain activity consistent with sleep with no elements of wakefulness. In humans, lesions along this pathway due to stroke, tumor, or other disease can result in lethargy and somnolence by interrupting the ascending reticular activating system. Examples of neuroanatomic locations where lesions result in lethargy and somnolence include the pons, midbrain, posterior hypothalamus, and thalamus.

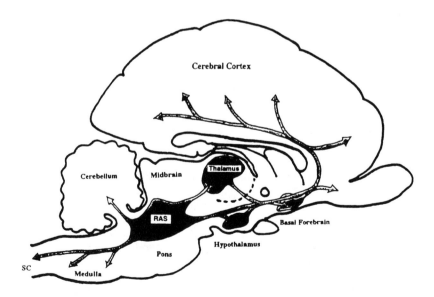

Figure 1. Ascending and descending reticular activating system (RAS) projections in a cat brain. Ascending pathways travel to the thalamus and activate the thalamocortical pathways. (From Garcia-Rill E: Mechanisms of sleep and wakefulness. In Lee-Chiong TL, Sateia MJ, Carskadon MA (eds): Sleep Medicine. Philadelphia, Hanley & Belfus, 2002, pp 31–39, with permission.)

3. Summarize the neurotransmitters that are thought to be involved in wakefulness and sleep, along with their site of release.

Neurotransmitters Involved in Wakefulness and Sleep

NEUROTRANSMITTER	SITE OF RELEASE
Wakefulness	
Norepinephrine*	Locus coeruleus and lateral tegmental area
Dopamine	Ventral tegmental area
Acetylcholine†	Basal forebrain, pedunculopontine tegmental nucleus, and latero-dorsal tegmental nuclei
Histamine	Posterior hypothalamus
Glutamate	Reticular formation and cortical projection neurons
Non–rapid-eye-movement (NREM) sleep	
Serotonin*	Dorsal raphe nucleus (midbrain, pons, medulla)
Adenosine	Present in extracellular region as degradation product of adenosine triphosphate (ATP)
	Hypothalamus and basal forebrain
	May be a neuromodulator that accumulates during wakefulness and enhances slow-wave sleep
Gamma-aminobutyric acid	Reticular formation, diencephalon, basal forebrain, hypothalamus, and thalamus (reticular nucleus)
Rapid-eye-movement (REM) sleep	
Acetylcholineᵗ	Basal forebrain, pedunculopontine tegmental nucleus, and latero-dorsal tegmental nuclei
Adenosine	Present in extracellular region as degradation product of adenosine triphosphate (ATP)
	Hypothalamus and basal forebrain
	May be a neuromodulator that accumulates during wakefulness and enhances slow-wave sleep

*Norepinephrine and serotonin are REM-off cells.
†Acetylcholine is a REM-on cell.

4. What neurotransmitters are thought to promote wakefulness?
Norepinephrine, dopamine, acetylcholine, histamine, and glutamate.

5. What pharmacologic evidence indicates that catecholamines promote wakefulness?
- Amphetamines, which promote wakefulness and result in arousal, increase the release of catecholamines, including dopamine and epinephrine.
- Cocaine induces alertness by preventing reuptake of the same catecholamines.
- Preparations that prevent the breakdown of catecholamines (such as monoamine oxidase inhibitors and catechol-o-methyltransferase) promote wakefulness.
- Preventing the synthesis of catecholamines by inhibiting crucial enzymes along the synthesis pathway (such as tyrosine hydroxylase) causes decreased wakefulness.
- Depletion of catecholamines with reserpine causes sedation.

6. Describe the pharmacologic action of acetylcholine.
Acetylcholine acts on two different receptors, muscarinic and nicotinic. Muscarinic receptors act through second-messenger systems (metabotropic), whereas nicotinic receptors act through direct links to ion channels (ionotropic). Cholinergic antagonists (e.g., atropine, belladonna) cause sedation, whereas cholinergic agonists (e.g., tobacco at nicotinic receptors) enhance alertness.

7. Where are the acetylcholine-producing cells located?

Neuroanatomic locations of acetylcholine-producing cells include the brainstem structures of the laterodorsal tegmental (LDT) nucleus and pedunculopontine nucleus (PPN) as well as the basal forebrain structures of the nucleus basalis, substantia innominata, and diagonal band nuclei.

8. How does histamine promote wakefulness?

Histamine neurons are located in the posterior hypothalamus, particularly the tuberomammillary nucleus (TMN), an anatomic structure important for its wake-promoting properties. This region is linked to cortical regions via the thalamocortical circuit, and activation results in wakefulness.

9. What is the most common practical implication of histamine's wake-promoting effect?

The most common practical implication is the sedation caused by antihistaminic allergy medication.

10. What other wake-promoting factors are found in cerebrospinal fluid (CSF) or blood?

Wake-promoting factors in the **CSF** may include substance P, corticotropin-releasing factor, thyrotropin-releasing factor, vasoactive intestinal peptide, and neurotensin. Wake-promoting factors contained in the **blood** include epinephrine, cortisol, histamine, corticotropin, and thyrotropin.

11. What neurotransmitters are thought to promote sleep?

Serotonin, adenosine, and gamma-aminobutyric acid (GABA).

12. What pharmacologic evidence supports the role of serotinin in promoting sleep?

Monoamine oxidase inhibitors used specifically to block the breakdown of serotonin result in increasing slow-wave sleep, whereas preventing synthesis of serotonin by blocking tryptophan hydroxylase results in insomnia.

13. What effect does caffeine have on adenosine receptors?

Caffeine (methylxanthine), which promotes alertness, blocks adenosine receptors. Agonists of adenosine increase slow-wave sleep, an effect blocked by caffeine. Adenosine accumulates during wakefulness, indicating a possible function as a sleep-inducing factor. Levels of adenosine decrease during sleep.

14. What major class of medications uses GABA receptors as the main mechanism of action?

Benzodiazepines bind to GABA receptors to enhance sleep. Other agents known to have their main mechanism of action through the GABA system include pentobarbital, gamma-hydroxybutyrate, and tiagabine.

15. What disorder has been shown to have elevated CSF concentrations of endozepine-4, a benzodiazepine-like factor? How are symptoms improved?

Idiopathic recurring stupor. Symptoms are improved by antagonism of benzodiazepine receptors.

16. What are the two different types of GABA receptors?

GABA-A receptors, the site of action for benzodiazepines, are linked to a chloride channel. GABA-B channels act through second-messenger systems and use potassium and calcium ion channels.

17. What CSF factors are thought to promote sleep?

Enkephalin, endorphin, dynorphin, alpha-melanocyte-stimulating hormone, somatostatin, growth hormone-releasing factor, prostaglandin D2, and interleukin.

18. What factors in the blood are thought to promote sleep?
Insulin, cholecystokinin, muramyl peptides, and delta sleep-inducing peptide.

19. Describe the pattern of the following neurotransmitters in wake, slow-wave sleep, and REM sleep: acetylcholine (Ach), norepinephrine (NE) and serotonin (SER).
Ach neurons are active both during wakefulness and REM sleep. NE and SER are active during wakefulness, but activity diminishes during NREM sleep. Both become even less active during REM sleep. The table below compares these different activities.

Neurotransmitters During Different States

NEUROTRANSMITTER	AWAKE	SLOW-WAVE SLEEP	REM SLEEP
Acetylcholine	+	−	+
Norepinephrine	+	+	−
Serotonin	+	+	−

20. Which part of the brain can generate REM sleep in transection studies?
Jouvet's studies in cats show that transection of the brainstem from the rest of the brain above the junction of the pons and midbrain generates periodic REM periods independently of the diencephalon and cortex.

21. Where are the REM-on neurons located?
The cholinergic systems of the laterodorsal tegmental nucleus (LDT) and the pedunculopontine nucleus (PPN) are considered REM-on neurons. As shown in Figure 2, REM-on neurons alternate with REM-off neurons in a cyclic fashion throughout the night.

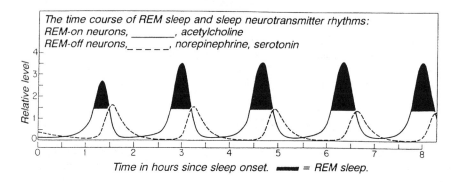

Figure 2. Cyclic relationship between the REM-on neurons and the REM-off neurons throughout the sleep cycle. (From McCarley RW: Sleep neurophysiology: Basic mechanisms underlying control of wakefulness and sleep. In Chokroverty S (ed): Sleep Disorders Medicine, 2nd ed. Boston, Butterworth-Heinemann, 1999, p 23, with permission.)

22. What neurotransmitters are associated with the REM-on state?
The cholinergic system has a strong influence on REM sleep. Acetylcholine is the neurotransmitter released from this system. The muscarinic receptors of the cholinergic system appear to be more relevant for REM sleep than the nicotinic receptors.

23. Where are the REM-off neurons located?
The REM-off neurons are located in the locus coeruleus, raphe nucleus, and posterior hypothalamus.

24. What neurotransmitters are associated with the REM-off state?

The adrenergic system, including norepinephrine and serotonin, is implicated for the REM-off state. In addition, histamine is considered REM-off. Figure 3 shows the activation of the reticular formation by the cholinergic REM-on neurons and the inhibition of REM sleep by REM-off neurons, which receive feedback from adenosine inhibition.

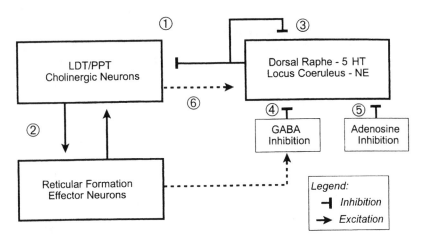

Figure 3. Interactions between the REM-on cholinergic neurons and REM-off aminergic neurons (5HT and NE). The cholinergic neurons activate the reticular formation to promote REM sleep. Feedback inhibition by adenosine and GABA help modulate REM-off neurons of the dorsal raphe and locus coeruleus. 5HT = serotonin. (From McCarley RW: Sleep neurophysiology: Basic mechanisms underlying control of wakefulness and sleep. In Sudhansu Chokroverty S (ed): Sleep Disorders Medicine, 2nd ed. Boston, Butterworth-Heinemann, 1999, p 35, with permission).

25. Where in the brain are norepinephrine, serotonin, and histamine produced?

Norepinephrine is produced in the locus coeruleus, serotonin in the raphe nucleus, and histamine in the posterior hypothalamus.

26. Which neuroanatomic pathway is responsible for the atonia of REM sleep?

The muscle atonia of REM is modulated by cells in the perilocus coeruleus region, which send excitatory signals via a pathway called the lateral tegmentoreticular tract to the reticularis magnocellularis nucleus of the medulla. The reticularis magnocellularis then sends a signal via a pathway called the ventrolateral reticulospinal tract, which hyperpolarizes spinal motorneuron cells.

27. What did Jouvet's studies reveal about the neuroanatomic basis for the atonia during REM sleep?

Jouvet's transection studies showed that bilateral ablation of the perilocus coeruleus region prevents the normal muscle atonia during REM sleep.

28. Where is the suprachiasmatic nucleus located? Describe its role in circadian rhythms.

The suprachiasmatic nucleus (SCN) is composed of paired nuclei located in the anterior hypothalamus dorsal to the optic chiasm. The retinohypothalamic tract sends input directly to the SCN to help modulate circadian rhythms.

29. How does the SCN influence secretion of melatonin from the pineal gland?

An efferent pathway from the SCN travels to the paraventricular nuclei (PVN) of the hypothalamus and subsequently to the intermediolateral (IML) horn of the spinal cord, which modulates the sympathetic nervous system by projecting to the superior cervical ganglion. The superior cervical ganglion directly links to the pineal gland and influences pineal release of melatonin. Melatonin release peaks during the night.

30. Which catecholamine is a precursor to the synthesis of melatonin?
Serotonin is a precursor to melatonin.

31. What is known about the neuroanatomy/neurophysiology of narcolepsy?
Recent studies have shed light on neuroanatomic and neurophysiologic abnormalities thought to cause narcolepsy. In certain canine breeds that genetically pass narcolepsy to their offspring, an abnormality was found in the receptor for hypocretin-2. Hypocretin, a protein made in the dorsolateral thalamus, promotes wakefulness. Pathologic studies of human narcoleptic brains show a dramatic reduction in the number of hypocretinergic neurons and gliosis in the dorsolateral hypothalamus. The etiology of this destruction is unclear, but one hypothesis proposes that it is immunologically mediated. The hypocretin system may be a target for future therapy for narcolepsy and offers further understanding of sleep and wakefulness.

32. How many neurons in the hypothalamus are responsible for making hypocretin?
The total number of neurons in the hypothalamus that are hypocretinergic is around 1500.

33. Where are hypocretins produced? What is their function?
Hypocretins are proteins that regulate wakefulness and sleep. In animal models and in reported cases of human narcoleptics with pathologic studies of the hypothalamus, the hypocretin system is dysfunctional. In dog models, the hypocretin-2 receptor is not functional. In human pathologic studies of narcoleptics, there is lack of neurons responsible for making hypocretin. In a subset of human narcoleptics (narcolepsy with cataplexy), CSF studies have shown abnormally absent or extremely low levels of hypocretin. The role of hypocretin in other sleep-wake disorders has yet to be established. The hypocretin system may be a target for future treatments of sleep disorders.

34. How does sleep affect the autonomic nervous system?
Parasympathetic tone predominates during NREM sleep. During REM sleep, tonic activity is mediated by parasympathetic tone, whereas phasic REM is the result of bursts of sympathetic tone.

35. What medullary nucleus is thought to be critical in integrating autonomic function?
Nucleus tractus solitarius.

36. What is the pupillary response during sleep?
The pupils become miotic during sleep with some pupillary size instability.

37. What are the three states of consciousness?
The three states of consciousness are NREM sleep, REM sleep, and wakefulness. Each has unique properties, although at times, particularly during disease states, they overlap.

38. What is the difference between NREM and REM sleep?
REM sleep is characterized by a highly active brain with recollection of dreams 80% of the time. NREM, on the other hand, is associated with reduced neuronal activity, and if patients recollect cognition, it is considered NREM cognition. NREM cognition typically is more reality-based and can involve ruminative thoughts but lacks the vivid visual accompaniment of REM sleep.

39. What is the behavioral definition of sleep?
Behaviorally, sleep is a reversible unconscious state with characteristic supine sleep posture, lack of mobility, closed eyes, and increased arousal threshold.

40. What is the neurophysiologic definition of sleep onset?

The polysomnographic definition of sleep onset is an electroencephalogram (EEG) in transition from the desynchronization with low-voltage waves and eye closure with predominantly alpha activity of wakefulness to greater than 50% of the epoch composed of a slowed pattern consisting of theta waves. Additional features include slow-rolling eye movements and decreased muscle tone.

41. Describe the EEG of wakefulness.

The EEG of wakefulness shows low-voltage, fast-frequency waves. This state is most similar to REM sleep.

42. What are the EEG characteristics of stage II sleep?

Stage II sleep is characterized by sleep spindles and K complexes on a background of predominantly theta waves. Sleep spindles have a frequency of 12–16 Hertz with a spindle appearance. K complexes show an initial downward deflection followed by an upward deflection, lasting at least 0.5 seconds followed by a spindle. Vertex waves last < 0.5 seconds and can be present during stage II sleep but are often seen during the later stages of stage I sleep.

43. What criteria are used to stage slow-wave sleep?

Slow-wave sleep is characterized by delta waves, which are defined by Rechtshaffen and Kales as 0.5- to 2-Hertz waves meeting an amplitude criterion of > 75 microvolts. Stage III is defined as 20–50% delta waves and stage 4 as > 50% delta waves.

44. What are the EEG criteria of REM sleep?

The EEG of REM sleep shows low-voltage, desynchronized rhythm with phasic eye movements and muscle atonia as measured by EMG. In animals, PGO (ponto-geniculo-occipital) spikes are seen as well. EEG characteristically shows saw-tooth waves, which are rhythmic waves in theta frequency maximal in the central leads.

45. In what stage of sleep are ponto-geniculo-occiptal (PGO) spikes seen?

PGO spikes are recorded from deeply placed electrodes in animal models during REM sleep.

46. What is the difference between tonic and phasic REM sleep?

Phasic REM is superimposed on tonic REM and is characterized by bursts of rapid eye movements, phasic twitches, PGO spikes, and irregular heart rate, breathing, and blood pressure indicating autonomic activation of the sympathetic nervous system. In addition, phasic REM shows spontaneous activity of the middle ear and tongue.

Tonic REM is the background activity during REM sleep with EEG patterns of low-voltage desynchronization, atonia of major muscles, and predominance of parasympathetic activity.

47. When does the first REM period typically occur?

The initial REM period occurs at the end of the first sleep cycle, approximately 70–120 minutes after sleep onset, depending on age and other factors.

48. What might a shortened REM latency indicate?

A shortened REM latency can be seen with depression, narcolepsy (typically less than 15 minutes), and withdrawal from REM-suppressing medications such as antidepressants or alcohol. In addition, REM latency may be short during recovery sleep as during continuous positive airway pressure (CPAP) titration and is considered "REM rebound."

49. At what time during the night is slow-wave sleep seen?

Slow-wave sleep is more prominent during the first one-third of the night.

50. At what time during the night is REM sleep most common?
REM sleep is more common during the last half of the night.

51. What happens to REM periods across the course of the night?
The REM periods progressively increase in length and phasic activity. Generally, 4–6 REM periods are seen across the course of the night in adult humans.

52. What percentage of a newborn's sleep is REM?
Newborns typically spend two-thirds of the 24 hours per day asleep, and half of that sleep is REM sleep.

53. Where are spindles generated in the brain?
Sleep spindles are generated in the reticular nucleus of the thalamus and are thought to "deafferent" or decrease afferent input into the cortex. In other words, spindles decrease external stimulation to the cortex, thereby facilitating sleep.

54. What is the frequency of different waves on EEG recordings?
The table below shows the frequency of the different waves. It should be noted that the delta frequency is different from the epileptologist's definition of 0.5–4 Hertz.

EEG Waves and Their Frequency

WAVE	FREQUENCY
Beta waves	16–25 Hertz
Alpha waves	8–12 Hertz
Theta waves	3–7 Hertz
Delta waves	0.5–2 Hertz

55. What maneuver during biocalibrations enhances alpha activity?
Eye closure typically enhances the occipitally predominant alpha activity. Alpha activity is seen more readily during relaxed wakefulness.

56. Which EEG leads best detect the delta waves of slow-wave sleep?
The delta waves of slow-wave sleep are more prominent in the frontal leads.

57. In which EEG leads are K complexes and spindles maximally seen?
K complexes and spindles are seen maximally in the central EEG leads.

58. Which EEG leads show alpha activity most prominently?
Alpha activity is more prominent in the occipital leads, although it can be transmitted to other leads.

59. At what age do spindles appear on the EEG?
Spindles are apparent on EEG at 3 months of age.

60. At what age do K complexes appear on the EEG?
K complexes appear at 6 months of age.

61. What percentage of total sleep in adults is composed of NREM?
NREM accounts for 75–80% of sleep time in adult humans.

62. What percentage of sleep in adults is composed of REM sleep?
REM sleep accounts for 20–25 % of total sleep time in adult humans.

63. What percentage of sleep in adults is composed of each of the NREM stages?
Stage I: 3–8%
Stage II: 45–55%
Stages III-IV: 15–20%

64. What happens to the distribution of the stages of sleep in the elderly population?
In the elderly population, there is a decrease in slow-wave sleep with a shift to lighter NREM sleep. REM sleep remains constant. In general, however, the elderly complain of more fragmented nighttime sleep and more time spent awake.

BIBLIOGRAPHY

1. Chokroverty S: Sleep Disorders Medicine, 2nd ed. Boston, Butterworth-Heinemann, 1999.
2. Jones BE: Basic mechanisms of sleep-wake state. In Kruger MH, Roth T, Dement WC: Principles and Practice of Sleep Medicine. Philadelphia, WB Saunders Company, 2000, pp 134–154.
3. Maquet P: Functional neuroimaging of normal human sleep by positron emission tomography. J Sleep Res Sep 9:207–231, 2000.
4. Rye DB: Contributions of the pedunculopontine region to normal and altered REM sleep. Sleep 20:757–788, 1997.
5. Tinton CM, McCarley RW: Neuroanatomical and neurophysiological aspects of sleep: Basic science and clinical relevance. Semin Clin Neuropsychiatry 5:6–19, 2000.
6. Tahert S, Zeitzer JM, Mignot E: The role of hypocretins (orexins) in sleep regulation and narcolepsy. Annu Rev Neurosci 25:283–313, 2002.

5. EVALUATION OF PATIENTS WITH SLEEP DISORDERS

Damien Stevens, MD

MEDICAL HISTORY

1. What important questions should be asked in evaluating patients with a sleep complaint?

The majority of patients evaluated for sleep disorders can be categorized as having excessive sleepiness or an inability to obtain adequate sleep. The majority of patients with excessive daytime sleepiness have insufficient sleep, sleep-disordered breathing, narcolepsy, or idiopathic hypersomnolence, whereas patients in the other group have insomnia, psychiatric disorders, or circadian disorders. Circadian disorders may also cause hypersomnolence. More rarely, patients may complain of abnormal nighttime behavior suggesting a parasomnia or sleep-wake transition disorder, although many of these patients also have hypersomnolence.

2. What important questions should be asked during the evaluation of patients for possible sleep-disordered breathing?

The best rule is to recall the risk factors for sleepapnea-hypopnea syndrome along with the most common symptoms and consequences of sleep apnea. The weight history, including a significant recent increase, is essential as well as a change in waist or neck circumference. Other changes in general health may also be a clue, such as a new thyroid disorder or cardiac dysfunction. A family history of snoring may suggest an anatomic or genetic link. The most common symptoms include loud snoring, witnessed apneas, nocturnal choking episodes, morning headaches, unrefreshing sleep, and excessive daytime sleepiness. Specific scales can be used for better assessment of daytime sleepiness but require more time to complete. Inquiring about recent motor vehicle, work-related, or other accidents related to daytime sleepiness should be done to avoid overlooking new potential injuries. The onset of symptoms varies greatly, but an acute onset should raise the possibility of a new coexistent process precipitating sleep apnea, such as partial upper airway obstruction from a tumor or neuromuscular disease with musculature compromise.

3. Why is a medication history critical in the evaluation of patients with a sleep complaint?

Medications can have a multitude of effects on sleep, but most commonly they affect the patients' sleepiness and wakefulness. More specifically, the four main effects include (1) insomnia, (2) daytime hypersomnolence, (3) suppression of rapid-eye-movement (REM) sleep, and (4) suppression of slow-wave sleep. In performing a multiple sleep latency test (MSLT), the effects of drugs of abuse, sedative/hypnotics, and REM-suppressant medications must be considered.

4. What is the Berlin Questionnaire for evaluation of sleep history?

The Berlin Questionnaire was developed as a screening test to evaluate patients for possible obstructive sleep apnea. As shown in Table 1, it includes a list of sleep-related symptoms, such as change in weight, snoring loudness and frequency, breathing pauses, sleepiness and fatigue, and the presence of hypertension. Responses to this questionnaire were grouped into different categories based on persistent snoring, daytime sleepiness, and hypertension or body mass index (BMI) more than 30 kg/m^2. High-risk patients include those who respond positively to at least two of the three categories. The questionnaire results in this high-risk group predicted an apnea-hypopnea index greater than 5 with a sensitivity of 86%, a specificity of 77%, a positive predictive value of 0.89, and a likelihood ratio of 3.79.

Table 1. *Berlin Questionnaire*

Has your weight changed?
Increased/ Decreased/ No change

Do you snore?
Yes/ No/ Do not know

Snoring loudness
Loud as breathing/ Loud as talking/ Louder than talking/ Very loud

Snoring frequency
Almost every day/ 3–4 times per week/ 1–2 times per week/ 1–2 times per month/ Never or almost never

Does your snoring bother other people?
Yes/ No

How often have your breathing pauses been noticed?
Almost every day/ 3–4 times per week/ 1–2 times per week/ 1–2 times per month/ Never or almost never

Are you tired after sleeping?
Almost every day/ 3–4 times per week/ 1–2 times per week/ 1–2 times per month/ Never or almost never

Are you tired during waketime?
Almost every day/ 3–4 times per week/ 1–2 times per week/ 1–2 times per month/ Never or almost never

Have you ever fallen asleep while driving?
Yes/ No

Do you have high blood pressure?
Yes/ No/ Do not know

From Netzer NC, et al: Using the Berlin Questionnaire to identity patients at risk for the sleep apnea syndrome. Ann Intern Med 131:485–491, 1999.

5. What is the Epworth Sleepiness Scale?

The Epworth Sleepiness Scale (Table 2) is one of the most widely used subjective methods to assess sleepiness. It is a short questionnaire that includes a list of 8 social circumstances with the likelihood that the person will fall asleep, rated on a 4-point scale. Patients rate the likelihood of dozing on a 0 to 3 scale: 0 = "would never doze," 1 = "slight chance of dozing," 2 = "moderate chance of dozing," and 3 = "high chance of dozing." The scale assesses probability of sleeping rather than specific feelings or symptoms of sleepiness. It usually has been shown to correlate with other objective measures of sleepiness such as the MSLT, although the correlation is typically weak. The maximum score is 24, and scores greater than 12 are thought to signify excessive daytime sleepiness. Normal subjects usually score less than 10.

Table 2. *Epworth Sleepiness Scale*

Sitting and reading
Watching TV
Sitting inactive in a public place (e.g., theater or a meeting)
As a passenger in a car for an hour without a break
Lying down to rest in the afternoon when the circumstances permit
Sitting and talking to someone
Sitting quietly after a lunch without alcohol
In a car, while stopped for a minute in traffic

From Johns MW: A new method for measuring sleepiness: The Epworth sleepiness scale. Sleep 14:540–545, 1991.

6. What is the Stanford Sleepiness Scale?

The Stanford Sleepiness Scale (Table 3) is another commonly used scale to assess sleepiness. It is a short questionnaire with several different responses used to describe the patient's current state of alertness rather than likelihood of dozing. The patient describes level of sleepiness on a 7-point scale according to his/her feelings and symptoms. This scale is limited in usefulness due to lack of reference values and validation of physiologic measures. On the other hand, it is probably more sensitive to the acute effects of sleep deprivation than the Epworth Sleepiness Scale and can be used repeatedly during an experimental sleep deprivation experiment.

Table 2. *Stanford Sleepiness Scale*

Feeling active and vital, alert; wide awake
Functioning at a high level, but not at peak: able to concentrate
Relaxed; awake; not at full alertness; responsive
A little foggy; not at peak; let down
Fogginess; beginning to lose interest in remaining awake; slowed down
Sleepiness; prefer to be lying down; fighting sleep; woozy
Almost in reverie; sleep onset soon; lost struggle to remain awake

From Glenville M, Broughton R: Reliability of the Stanford Sleepiness Scale compared to short duration performance tests and the Wilkinson Auditory Vigilance Task. Adv Biosci 21:235-244, 1978.

7. What other scales are available to assess sleepiness?

- The Karolinska Sleep Institute developed a short questionnaire as a measure of sleepiness known as the Karolinska Sleepiness Scale.
- The Sleep-Wake Activity Inventory consists of 35 items. One subscale assesses sleepiness, and results appear to be similar to those of the Epworth Sleepiness Scale.
- A visual analog scale also has been used. The patient designates degree of alertness-sleepiness on a 10-cm scale. This test is obviously one of the most simple, but there is no consensus about the "best" subjective test for sleepiness.

8. What important questions should be asked during the history in evaluating patients for insomnia?

The date of onset of insomnia is one of the most critical questions. Typically patients with a longer history of insomnia have a poorer prognosis and a more complicated history. Precipitating factors should be sought, such as a change in financial or social circumstances. Any prior treatment regimens should be reviewed, including medications, alterations in sleep patterns or nighttime routine, and whether there is improvement or resolution of the insomnia during travel or vacation (suggesting psychophysiologic insomnia). Assessments of the patient's bedtime, awake time, total time spent in bed, number of arousals, and time to fall asleep or back to sleep should also be noted. An inquiry should be made into the patient's general health and any new medications since many medical disorders and medications may be associated with insomnia. Special attention should be paid to possible psychiatric disorders such as depression, panic, or anxiety.

9. What important questions should be asked during the history in evaluating patients with epilepsy and a potential sleep disorder?

Up to 20% of patients with epilepsy have seizures mainly during sleep, and up to 30% have at least some seizures during sleep. However, these percentages can vary widely, depending on the type of seizure. Seizure activity is usually not subtle, but in some patients more complex motor activity may be present. In such cases, differentiating a frontal lobe seizure from sleepwalking or other parasomnia may not be so straightforward.

10. What historical questions are important in evaluating a patient for possible REM behavior disorder?

Patients with REM behavior disorder specifically display dream-enacting behavior and typically recall specific dreams.

11. What historical questions are important in differentiating NREM from REM parasomnias?

Patients with NREM parasomnia typically do not recall dreams or appear to act out dreams. Patients with REM behavior disorder typically display more complex behavior than patients with NREM disorders.

12. How is a sleep terror different from a nightmare, based on the patient's history?

Sleep terrors usually occur during slow-wave sleep or delta sleep, whereas nightmares usually occur during REM sleep. Because slow-wave sleep is more prevalent earlier in the sleep period, sleep terrors typically occur earlier in the night; because REM sleep occurs later in the sleep period, nightmare are more common in the early morning hours. However, these are only "rules of thumb" because patients go through all stages of sleep both early and late in the sleep period.

13. What important questions should be asked in evaluating patients for possible narcolepsy?

Hypersomnolence, sleep paralysis, cataplexy, and hypnagogic or hypnopompic hallucinations are considered the cardinal symptoms or tetrad of narcolepsy. Hypersomnolence typically develops first (but not in all patients), and obviously there are multiple causes of hypersomnolence. In addition, up to 50% of healthy people report sleep paralysis at least once in their life. Cataplexy is strongly suggestive of narcolepsy, but occasionally normal patients develop a vague weakness associated with emotional triggers. Hypnagogic hallucinations occur at sleep onset, whereas hypnopompic hallucinations occur during waking. These hallucinations are most often visual or auditory, but tactile hallucinations may also occur. Again, these symptoms can occur in otherwise normal people.

14. What important questions should be asked in evaluating patients for possible parasomnias?

Major questions are what type of behavior is displayed and how complex the behavior is. Other questions should focus on whether the behavior is stereotypical and/or aggressive and whether it varies from night to night. Another clue is the time of night during which the behavior is displayed. Slow-wave sleep is predominantly earlier during the sleep period, whereas REM sleep is more common later during the sleep period. Whether a patient recalls the behavior is a useful question because certain parasomnias are associated with recall. The childhood sleep history and family history may suggest certain sleep disorders. Current stressors, sleep hygiene, and sleep sufficiency should be reviewed because all of these factors may be associated with some parasomnias.

PHYSICAL EXAMINATION

15. What are the critical vital signs in patients evaluated for sleep apnea-hypopnea syndrome (SAHS)?

Most are the same as for all other patients undergoing a medical evaluation. Blood pressure is important to evaluate the possible presence of hypertension. Oxygen saturation may reveal the unsuspected presence of hypoxemia. Fluctuations during oximetry recording may suggest Cheyne-Stokes or periodic breathing, but prolonged oximetry rather than a quick oxygen saturation "spot check" may be required to uncover this finding. Height and weight are obviously important because they allow the calculation of body mass index (BMI), which is one of the strongest predictors of SAHS. BMI is the weight in kilograms divided by the square of the height in meters. Neck circumference is a weak predictor of SAHS, although measurements greater than 18 inches in men and 16 inches in women correlate with the presence of SAHS.

16. What are the important parts of the physical examination in patients evaluated for sleep-disordered breathing?

The physical examination of patients evaluated for sleep-disordered breathing should typically focuses on certain organ systems. An upper airway examination is essential, including the nasal and oral cavity. The nares should be examined to exclude obstruction, rhinitis, polyps, or inflammation since treatment for these conditions may be required for further diagnosis or before treatment is undertaken. Oropharyngeal examination is essential to evaluate for evidence of anatomic contributions to sleep-disordered breathing, such as a low-lying palate, large tongue, enlarged tonsils, or craniofacial abnormalities. The cardiopulmonary examination is important to detect any cardiac or lung disease that may predispose patients to sleep-disordered breathing. Cardiac examination should focus on signs of heart failure since Cheyne-Stokes respirations or central sleep apnea may be associated findings. The neurologic examination may reveal a central nervous system or neuromuscular condition, which may also contribute to sleep-disordered breathing, both central and obstructive.

17. How good is a physical examination for the diagnosis of SAHS?

One study evaluated the performance of physical examination and history in screening patients suspected of SAHS. The investigators found that in patients with a low predicted probability of SAHS, the sensitivity of their model was 94% and the specificity was 28%. Subjective impression alone in patients with a high predicted probability of SAHS identified only 52% of patients correctly. The authors concluded that a significant number of sleep studies can be avoided but only in patients with a low index of suspicion for SAHS.

18. What are the important parts of the physical examination in patients with neurologic diseases who are evaluated for a sleep disorder?

To a large degree the answer depends on the patient's specific sleep complaint. Symptoms of nocturnal hypoventilation, such as morning headaches or pedal edema due to secondary cor pulmonale, raise the possibility of neuromuscular disorders. An evaluation of muscle strength and reflexes, including observation for fasciculations, is essential. Patients with a history consistent with REM-behavior disorder should be carefully examined for signs of parkinsonism, including observation for rest tremor, bradykinesia, and postural instability.

19. How is the Muller maneuver performed? What value does it have in evaluating patients with sleep-disordered breathing?

The Muller maneuver consists of a forceful inspiration while the glottis or vocal cords are closed. Originally thought to predict obstructive sleep apnea or even the response to upper airway surgery, the Muller maneuver has since been shown to be a poor predictor for either outcome.

20. What airway classification system is used to designate the degree of posterior pharyngeal crowding?

The modified Mallampati classification system (Fig. 1) is the most common system used to categorize the severity of posterior pharyngeal crowing. It was originally developed to predict difficult tracheal intubation but has been commonly used to assess and classify upper airway patency. The patient is asked to open the mouth fully but without protrusion of the tongue. The

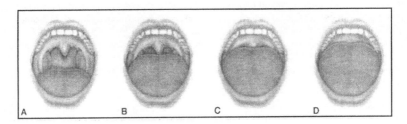

Figure 1. Modified Mallampati airway classification system. A, Mallampati I; B, Mallampati II; C, Mallampati III; D, Mallampati IV. (From Friedman M, et al: Clinical predictors of obstructive sleep apnea. Laryngoscope 109:1901-1907, 1999, with permission.)

airway is categorized from 1 to 4, depending on how much of the airway orifice is visible. Basically, the entire uvula and tonsils/pillars are visualized in class I airways; the uvula but not the tonsils is visualized in class II airways; the soft palate but not the uvula is visualized in class III airways; and only the hard palate is visible in class IV airways. The modified Mallampati class has been shown to be a weak predictor of the presence of SAHS.

21. How is the degree of tonsillar enlargement reported?
Tonsils are classified from grade 0 to grade IV based on the degree of enlargement (Fig. 2). Grade 1 tonsils are hidden by the pillars, grade 2 tonsils extend past the pillars; grade 3 tonsils extend pass the pillars but do not reach the midline; and grade 4 tonsils extend to the midline. Tonsil size has been shown to correlate with the presence of SAHS, but it is a very weak predictor.

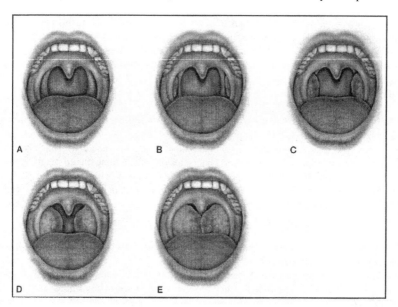

Figure 2. Tonsil grades. A, grade 0; B, grade I; C, grade II; D, grade III; E, grade IV. (From Friedman M, et al: Clinical predictors of obstructive sleep apnea. Laryngoscope 109:1901-1907, 1999, with permission.)

BIBLIOGRAPHY

1. Aldrich MS: Approach to the patient. In Aldrich MS (ed): Sleep Medicine. New York, Oxford University Press, 1999, pp 95-110.
2. Fairbanks DNF: Snoring: A general overview with historical perspective. In Fairbanks DNF, Mickelson SA, Woodson BT (eds): Snoring and Obstructive Sleep Apnea, 3rd ed. Philadelphia, Lippincott Williams & Wilkins, 2003, pp 1-17.
3. Mysliwiec V, Henderson JH, Strollo PJ: Epidemiology, consequences, and evaluation of excessive daytime sleepiness. In Teofilo LLC, Sateia M, Carskadon MA (eds): Sleep Medicine. Philadelphia, Hanley & Belfus, 2002, pp 187-192.

6. POLYSOMNOGRAPHY

Suzanne Stevens, MD, and Glenn Clark, RPSGT

1. What is a polysomnogram?

A polysomnogram (PSG) is a test consisting of electroencephalography (EEG), electro-oculography (EOG), electromyography (EMG), electrocardiography (ECG or EKG), and data from various ancillary monitors of respiratory effort and airflow, blood oxygen saturation, and audiovisual recording. The use of digital signal processing and analysis allows collection of virtually any number of biologic processes or physical activity that can be converted into an alternating or direct voltage potential.

INDICATIONS

2. What sleep disorders require polysomnography for diagnosis?

PSG is routinely indicated for the diagnosis of sleep-related breathing disorders (both obstructive and central sleep apneas) and periodic limb movement disorder. PSG is also commonly performed during titration of continuous positive airway pressure (CPAP), preoperative evaluation before upper airway surgery for snoring, and follow-up after certain treatment modalities.

3. What are the indications for polysomnography in patients with insomnia?

PSG is indicated when symptoms of insomnia are not adequately diagnosed by obtaining a sleep history, assessing sleep hygiene, and reviewing sleep diaries.

4. When is polysomnography indicated in patients with parasomnias?

PSG with extended EEG channels is indicated when sleep disruption is thought to be seizure-related. PSG is indicated in evaluating sleep-related behaviors that are violent or injurious, unusual or atypical for the parasomnia in question, or when data need to be collected and analyzed for forensic purposes.

5. Why is the constant presence of a trained professional required for polysomnography?

The trained professional monitors for technical quality, patient compliance, and relevant patient behaviors.

ELECTROENCEPHALOGRAPHY

6. How is the position of the EEG electrodes determined?

The placement of the EEG electrodes is based on the International 10-20 System. The landmarks are the **nasion** (the bridge of the nose at the forehead), the **inion** (the occipital protuberance), and the **preauricular point** (the bony indentation in front of the ear). Measurements are made from the nasion to the inion with Fp marked at 10% posterior to the nasion. Fz, Cz, and Pz are each 20% of the distance behind Fpz. The distance between the two preauricular points is also measured, with C3 and C4 each being 20% from the center and with T3 and T4 40% from the midline. Lastly, the circumference is measured, including the occipital point (10% anterior to the inion), T3, and T4 as well as Fp1. This set-up is shown in Figure 1.

7. Why and how are biocalibrations performed?

Figure 2 shows a typical biocalibration procedure. Biocalibration assesses eye movements, the EEG waveforms (alpha frequency should increase with eye closure), chin EMG, airflow and chest/abdominal excursion with inspiration, and leg movements to ensure that the channels are recording appropriately.

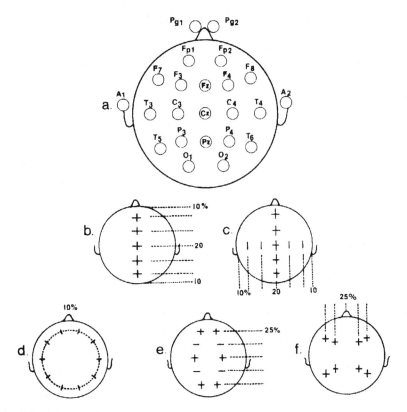

Figure 1. The placement of recording electrodes for an EEG by the International 10-20 System. The letters represent the following: frontopolar (Fp), frontal (F), central (C), parietal (P), occipital (O), and auricular (A). Lower case z indicates midline, odd numbers indicate left side, and even numbers indicate right side. The reference points for placement of the electrodes are the nasion (bridge of the nose), the inion (bony protuberance in the back of the head), and the preauricular point (bony depression in front of the ear). (From Fisch BJ: Spehlmann's EEG Primer, 2nd ed. Amsterdam, Elsevier Science, 1991, p 32, with permission.)

8. What are the different parts of an EEG recording?

Figure 3 shows the different steps and components of a paper EEG recording. Basically, it consists of a source, an input board, amplifiers, filters, a writing unit, and the actual tracing. With newer computerized systems the files are recorded without producing a paper tracing.

9. Describe the different filters and settings for a PSG recording.

Frequency filters are set according to the signal that the investigator desires to measure, since each signal gives meaningful data only within a certain range of hertz (Hz). For the EEG, the low-frequency filter is set at 0.3 Hz (cycles per second), and the high-frequency filter is set at 30–35 Hz. EMG uses a low-frequency filter of 10 Hz and a high-frequency filter of 63 Hz.

10. What are the effects of different filters on the recorded waveform?

The 60-hertz filter or notch filter is used when the examiner needs to decrease artifact from electrical sources. However, it can also filter out physiologic activity, such as chin EMG muscle tone and epileptiform discharges. The effects of changing low and high filter settings as well as using the 60-hertz filters are shown in Figure 4.

11. Define sensitivity as it pertains to electroencephalography.

Sensitivity is defined as the voltage divided by the pen deflection.

12. What is meant by the time constant?

The time constant is generated by delivering a voltage source and assessing the time required for the voltage to rise by 63% and drop to 37% of its amplitude (Fig. 5). The most commonly used time constant settings range between 1 and 0.03 seconds. An increase in the time constant means that waves of lower frequency are amplified without distortion.

13. What are epochs?

An epoch of a PSG has traditionally been defined as a 30-second page or screen of data. This is the basic "unit" or page used in analyzing and reporting PSG data.

14. What EEG activities and frequencies are encountered in a PSG?
- Beta: > 16 hertz
- Alpha: 8-12 hertz
- Theta: 3-7 hertz
- Delta: < 2 hertz (defined in epileptology as < 4 hertz)

15. Which EEG leads are commonly monitored in a PSG?

Although any number of leads and montages can be used, most PSG recordings routinely monitor central leads (C3 and C4) and occipital leads (O1 and O2). By the Rechtschaffen and Kales scoring manual, only the central lead is necessary for scoring.

16. Why are eye movements monitored in a PSG?

There are characteristic slow-roving eye movements at sleep onset and rapid eye movements throughout rapid-eye-movement (REM) sleep. Figure 6A shows typical rapid eye movements.

17. What type of eye movements typically heralds the onset of sleep?

Slow, roving eye movements, as shown in Figure 6B, often occur with drowsiness and stage I sleep.

18. Which muscle is typically monitored for an EMG lead during PSG?

By monitoring the mentalis/submentalis (chin) muscles, changes in EMG activity can be seen as non-REM deepens and most notably during the atonia associated with REM sleep. EMG activity of the anterior tibialis muscles is also routinely monitored for diagnosing periodic limb movement disorder (PLMD).

19. What anatomic structure generates spindles?

The reticular nucleus of the thalamus.

20. In which EEG leads are spindles more prominent?

Spindles are more prominent in the central EEG leads.

21. Define the K complex.

The K complex is a diphasic waveform with a slow, negative (upward) EEG waveform, immediately followed by a positive (downward) component. It is commonly followed by a spindle or burst of alpha (known as K alpha). An example of a K complex is shown in Figure 7.

22. Describe the EEG of stage I sleep.

Low-voltage, mixed-frequency EEG activity comprising more than 50% of an epoch defines stage I sleep.

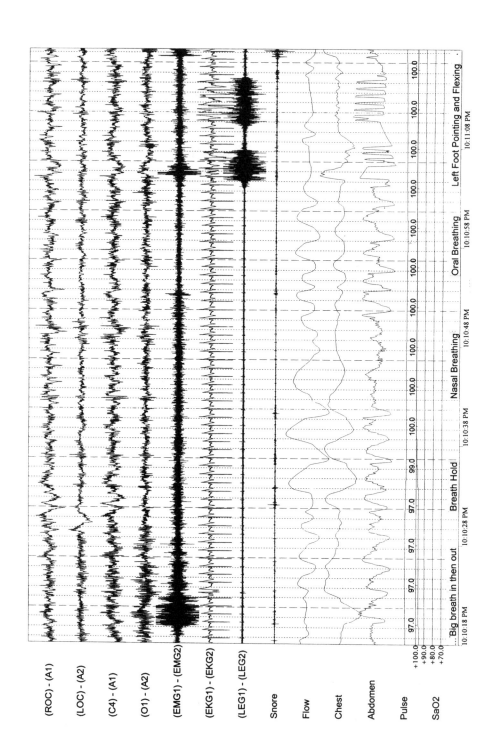

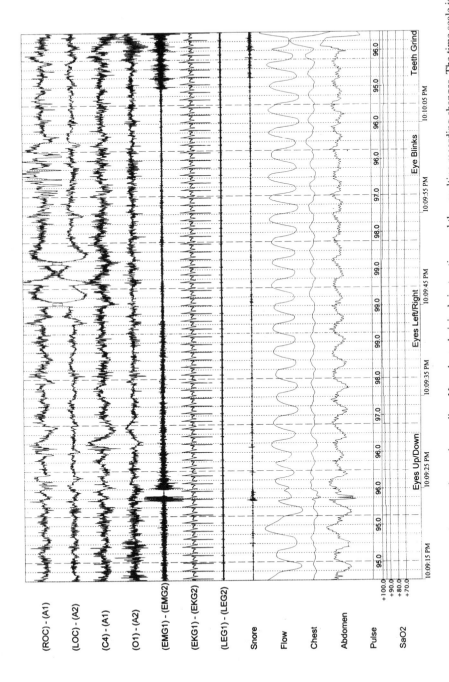

Figure 2. *A* and *B,* Typical biocalibration procedure and recording. Note the technician's instructions and the resulting recording changes. The time scale is 60 seconds per epoch.

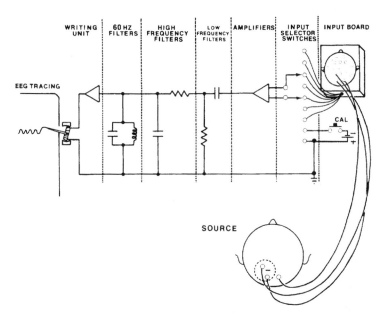

Figure 3. EEG electrodes on the scalp record the electrical differences between the two sites being transferred to the amplifier through the input board and input selector switches. From this point, the signal passes through low- and high-frequency filters as well as other set filters (e.g., notch filter) as it finishes in the recording unit. (From Fisch BJ: Spehlmann's EEG Primer, 2nd ed. Amsterdam, Elsevier Science, 1991, p 4 with permission.)

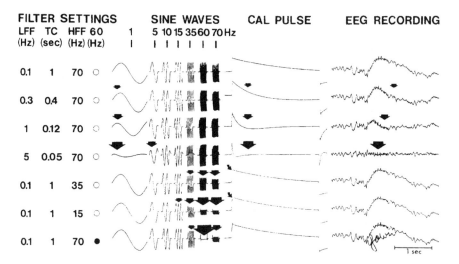

Figure 4. The effect of different filters and time constant settings on EEG waveforms. The first four examples show the effect of progressively increasing the low filter setting, which eliminates the waveform produced by yawning. The next two examples show the effect of decreasing the high filter, which eliminates the fast waveforms, whereas the slower waveform produced by yawning persists. The final example shows the effects of a 60-hertz filter (i.e., notch filter). (Fisch BJ: Spehlmann's EEG Primer, 2nd ed. Amsterdam, Elsevier Science, 1991, p 52, with permission.)

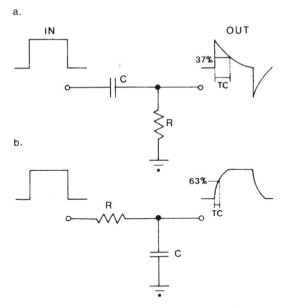

Figure 5. The waveform of the time constant, which is generated by delivering a voltage source and assessing the time required for the voltage to rise by 63% and drop to 37% of its amplitude. C = capacitance; R = resistor; TC = time constant. (From Fisch BJ: Spehlmann's EEGj Primer, 2nd ed. Amsterdam, Elsevier Science, 1991, p. 56, with permission.)

23. What is a sleep spindle?
Spindles display a frequency of 12–16 hertz. Their shape has been compared with a full or empty spinning-wheel thread spindle, with paired increasing/decreasing or decreasing/increasing amplitudes An example of a spindle is shown in Figure 8.

24. In which stage of sleep are spindles and K complexes typically seen?
Spindles and K complexes usually are seen in stage II sleep. However, they can be seen in stage III sleep as well.

25. What percentage of delta must be present to define stage III sleep?
Between 20% and 50% of an epoch must be delta sleep to be defined as stage III sleep.

26. What percentage of delta must be present to define stage IV sleep?
Greater than 50% of an epoch must be delta sleep to be defined as stage IV sleep.

27. In which EEG leads is alpha activity more prominent?
The occipital leads. Alpha activity is shown in Figure 9.

28. What maneuver enhances alpha activity?
Eye closure.

29. In which EEG leads is delta more prominent?
Delta is more prominent in the central and frontal leads.

30. What are vertex waves?
Vertex waves are well-delineated, sharp, negative waves typically occurring during the latter stages of stage I sleep. They are more prominent over the central leads.

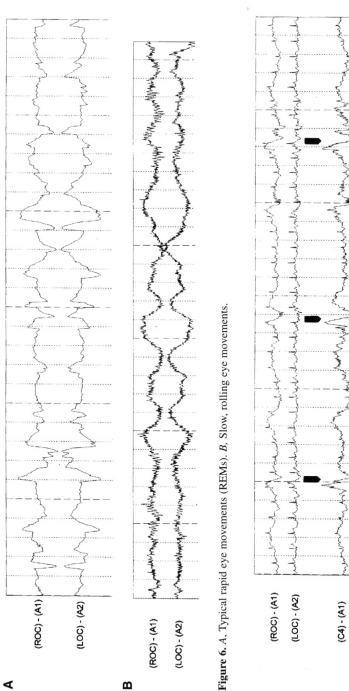

Figure 6. *A*, Typical rapid eye movements (REMs). *B*, Slow, rolling eye movements.

Figure 7. Typical K complexes, designated by arrows.

31. What type of background EEG accompanies REM sleep?

Low-voltage, mixed-frequency background EEG accompanies REM sleep.

32. In which stage of sleep are saw-tooth waves seen?

Saw-tooth waves are seen during REM sleep. They are repetitive, theta in frequency, with well-delineated positive and negative components of equivalent height or amplitude (like the teeth of a saw). Saw-tooth waves are more prominent in the central leads. An example of a saw-tooth wave is shown in Figure 10.

33. What features define REM sleep?

Rapid eye movements, absent chin tone, and saw-tooth waves on a low-voltage, mixed-frequency EEG.

RESPIRATORY MEASUREMENTS

34. How can respiratory effort be assessed during polysomnography?

Many ways of monitoring respiratory effort have been used, including intercostal EMG, mercury-filled tube strain gauges, piezo-crystal accelerimetry, and respiratory inductance plethysmography.

35. Is the nasal transducer accurate for assessing respiratory effort?

The nasal transducer is a fairly new method of measuring respiratory effort. In clinical trials, it appears to be more sensitive in picking up respiratory events than EMG, strain gauges, and inductance plethysmography. It also has been compared with esophageal manometry in several studies. Once again, it seems to have a fairly high sensitivity, picking up most events recorded by esophageal balloon, and a very high specificity.

36. What is the gold standard for assessing respiratory effort?

There is no universally accepted gold standard for assessing respiratory effort, but most physiologists agree than an esophageal balloon is the most accurate method for assessing the effort to breathe. Since esophageal pressure, when measured accurately, reflects pleural pressure, deflections represent effort. The esophageal balloon may be even more relevant in patients with neuromuscular disease, who may have weak efforts that are not picked up by measures other than esophageal manometry. The downside to esophageal manometry is that an esophageal balloon obviously affects sleep quality and continuity.

37. Why are both respiratory airflow and respiratory effort monitored?

Apneas and hypopneas are defined by the change in airflow, but the type or cause of the sleep-disordered breathing is defined by comparing airflow with effort.

38. Why are both thoracic and abdominal efforts monitored?

Paradoxical breathing is seen when the airway closes off during apneas and respiratory effort continues. Physiologically, the thorax expands with abdominal contraction, followed by abdominal expansion with thoracic contraction.

39. What is an obstructive apnea?

Obstructive apneas occur when the airway closes off and respiratory effort continues.

40. What is a central apena?

Central apneas occur when respiratory effort ceases, leading to absence of airflow.

41. What is a mixed apnea?

Mixed apneas occur when respiratory effort ceases, the airway collapses, and respiratory efforts begin again against the obstructed airway. Most mixed apneas appear as a central apnea followed by an obstructive apnea.

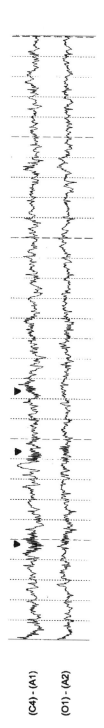

(C4) - (A1)

(O1) - (A2)

Figure 8. Typical spindle activity, designated by arrows.

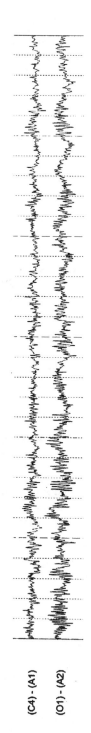

(C4) - (A1)

(O1) - (A2)

Figure 9. Typical alpha activity. Note that the activity is more prominent in the occipital lead than in the central lead.

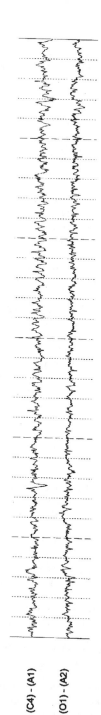

(C4) - (A1)

(O1) - (A2)

Figure 10. Typical saw-tooth waves as seen during REM sleep. Note that they are more prominent in the central lead than in the occipital lead.

42. Define hypopnea.

The actual definition of hypopnea is widely debated. One definition is any decrease in air-flow associated with an arousal or desaturation of blood oxygen.

43. How is blood oxygen saturation monitored?

Oxygen saturation in arterial blood (SpO_2) is usually recorded via a finger pulse oximeter, which utilizes chromospectroscopy. Two frequencies of red and infrared light are shown through a patient's finger. The oximeter calculates the percent saturation according to how much light is absorbed by the oxygenated/deoxygenated hemoglobins in the blood.

44. What other ancillary equipment has been used during PSGs? Why?

Equipment	Indication
Nasogastric esophageal pH probes	Gastroesophageal reflux
Mercury strain gauges	Nocturnal penile tumescence
Finger/wrist plethysmography	Frequent blood pressure monitoring
Galvanic skin response	Arousal/response to stimuli
Arterial blood catheter	Drawing of arterial blood gases
Transcranial oximeter	Cerebral oxygenation
Suprasternal notch pressure monitor	Upper airway resistance syndrome
Ankle/foot accelerimetry	PLMD/restless legs syndrome
Rectal temperature probe	Core body temperature
Sound decibel meter	Snoring

45. What recording montage, sensitivity, and filter settings are typically used for a polysomnogram?

Sample Recording Montage: Nocturnal Polysomnogram

Channel	Derivation	Sensitivity	Low-frequency Filter (TC)	High-frequency Filter	60-Hz Filter
1	C3/A2 or C4/A1	50 µV/cm	0.3 Hz (0.25 sec)	30–35 Hz	Off
2	O2/A1 or O1/A2	50 µV/cm	0.3 Hz (0.25 sec)	30–35 Hz	Off
3	ROC/A1	50 µV/cm	0.3 Hz (0.25 sec)	30–35 Hz	Off
4	LOC/A2	50 µV/cm	0.3 Hz (0.25 sec)	30–35 Hz	Off
5	Chin EMG	50 µV/cm	10 Hz (0.01 sec)	90–100 Hz	Off
6	Right leg EMG	50 µV/cm	10 Hz (0.01 sec)	90–100 Hz	On (if needed)
7	Left leg EMG	50 µV/cm	10 Hz (0.01 sec)	90–100 Hz	On (if needed)
8	ECG	1 mV/cm	1 Hz (0.1 sec)	30–35 Hz	Off
9	Nasal/oral flow	Variable	0.1 Hz (1 sec)	0.5 Hz	Off
10	Chest wall movement	Variable	0.1 Hz (1 sec)	0.5 Hz	Off
11	Abdominal movement	Variable	0.1 Hz (1 sec)	0.5 Hz	Off
12	Oximetry	I V/F cm	DC	15 Hz	Off

TC = time constant.
From School of Clinical Polysomnography, Medford, OR.

POLYSOMNOGRAM PARAMETERS

46. What is latency to sleep onset?

Length of time in minutes from "lights out" to the first epoch of sleep.

47. What is a normal sleep latency?

Normal, well-rested people typically take from 15 to 20 minutes to fall asleep. However, few studies have reported normal values in large populations, and sleep latency appears to be longer for laboratory studies compared with home studies.

48. What is latency to persistent sleep?
The length of time from "lights out" until a certain number of consecutive epochs of sleep, usually 6 or 10 epochs (3–5 minutes). This parameter discounts the brief or transient periods of sleep as the subject dozes.

49. What is REM latency?
Length of time in minutes from sleep onset to the first epoch of REM sleep. Note that this time period is measured from sleep onset and not from "lights out."

50. What is a normal REM latency?
A normal, healthy person has an REM latency of 90–120 minutes.

51. What is time in bed (TIB)?
The total time of data collection from "lights out" to "lights on."

52. What is total sleep time (TST)?
The sum of all minutes spent in all stages of sleep, or the TIB minus all time spent awake during the study.

53. What is sleep efficiency?
The total sleep time divided by the time in bed, multiplied by 100. The equation is TST/(TIB × 100).

54. How is the amount of each sleep stage reported?
Because the length of studies varies, the actual number of minutes of each sleep stage is difficult to compare between studies and subjects. Therefore, the percentage of each sleep stage is typically reported. The equation is (X minutes of stage Y/TST) × 100 = percentage stage Y.

55. Why are stages III and IV often combined?
Because the difference between stage III and stage IV is an arbitrary percent of delta activity and no clinical significance has been found between the amount of stage III vs. the amount of stage IV sleep, this parameter is frequently reported as stage III/IV or delta sleep. In addition, inter-rater reliability is poor in distinguishing stage III from stage IV sleep.

56. What is an arousal?
Although consensus criteria are now available for scoring arousals, a working definition of an arousal is an increase in EEG and/or EMG activity (frequency and amplitude) that varies significantly from the background activity defining the current sleep stage. Arousals often herald a change in sleep stage.

57. How are arousals reported on a PSG?
Arousals are totaled for the entire study and reported as an index—that is, a number of arousals per hour of total sleep time. Arousal index = number of arousals/hours of TST. Arousal data are commonly broken down into categories based on the probable cause of the arousal (e.g., respiratory, periodic limb movements, idiopathic). It must be noted that the specific cause of the arousal is not always evident.

58. What are periodic limb movements?
Periodic limb movements (PLMs) occur in clusters of at least four bursts. Each individual burst lasts 0.5–5 seconds, and bursts occur at intervals between 4 and 90 seconds. PLMs have also been called nocturnal myoclonus.

59. How are PLMs reported on a PSG?

PLMs that meet the criteria in question 58 are counted as individual bursts and reported as an index, or number of PLMs per hour. PLM index = number of PLMs/hours of TST. PLM data are often broken down into two categories: with and without associated EEG arousals.

60. How are respiratory events reported on a PSG?

Respiratory events are reported in a respiratory distress index (RDI), also known as an apnea/hypopnea index (AHI). RDI = number of events/hours of TST. AHI is often broken down into an apnea index, hypopnea index, events with arousals, events with desaturations of oxygen, and events in REM versus NREM sleep. In addition, position is important because some people have purely positional obstructive sleep apnea while in the supine position.

61. What is first-night effect?

First-night effect is defined as the combined effects of having monitors attached, sleeping in a different environment, and being watched. Sleep onset latency, REM latency, and the amount of wake after sleep onset (WASO) may increase during the first night in the sleep laboratory compared with subsequent nights. The first-night effect needs to be taken into consideration during interpretation of data, raw and derived.

62. What is an artifact?

Artifacts are signals or data that do not actually represent the biologic or physical phenomena that one wishes to measure. Artifacts can be superimposed over interpretable data or totally obscure the data being collected.

63. List and describe common sources of artifacts.
- 60-hertz ambient electrical activity: high-frequency "buzz" of constant amplitude
- Muscle activity in EMG leads: high-frequency activity of variabe amplitude
- Electrode "popping": fast, high-amplitude activity of short duration
- Sweat under electrode: slow (< 1 hertz), rolling waves obscuring data
- Respiratory artifact: slow, rolling waves due to respiratory effort
- EKG artifact: fast "pulse" corresponding to EKG
- Ballistocardiogram: "pulsating" waves due to cardiac contractions

Examples of these artifacts are shown in Figures 11–16.

64. What can be done to diminish the effect of artifacts on a PSG?

For fast activity, the high-frequency filter may be lowered. For slow activity, the low-frequency filter may be raised. For 60-hertz interference, a notch filter may be applied. However, adjusting filters has the undesired effect of obscuring or eliminating the actual data that one may wish to collect.

65. How can artifacts be eliminated?

Often especially in montages with redundant leads, substituting another input lead for the artifact-affected lead is advisable. In addition, re-referencing to a similar lead can eliminate artifact. For many environmental artifacts, the best solution is to find and eliminate the source. Replacing, repairing, re-prepping, and reattaching leads properly may eliminate or reduce many artifacts.

BIBLIOGRAPHY

1. Butkov N: Atlas of Clinical Polysomnography. Ashland, OR, Synapse Media, 1996.
2. Fisch BJ: Spehlmann's EEG Primer, 2nd ed. Amsterdam, Elsevier Science, 1991.
3. Rechtschaffen A, Kales A: A Manual of Standardized Terminology, Techniques, and Scoring System for the Sleep Stages of Human Subjects. Los Angeles, UCLA BIS/BRI Publications, 1968.

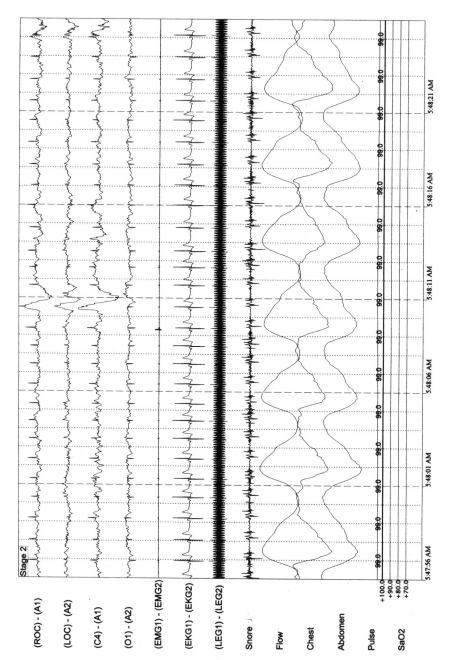

Figure 11. Typical 60-hertz artifact seen in (LEG1) – (LEG2) before application of a 60-hertz or notch filter.

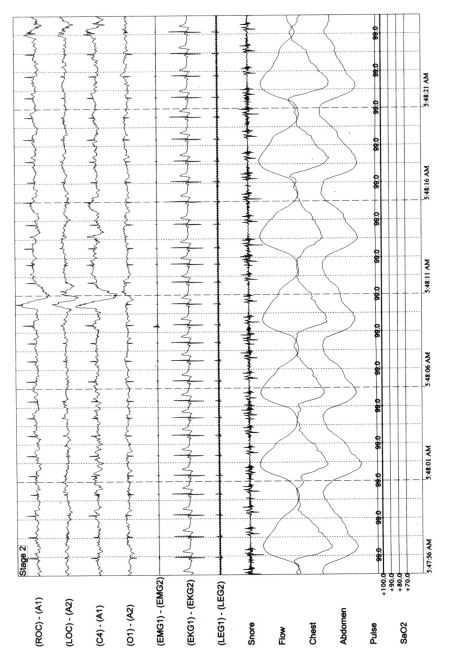

Figure 12. Typical 60-hertz artifact after application of a 60-hertz or notch filter.

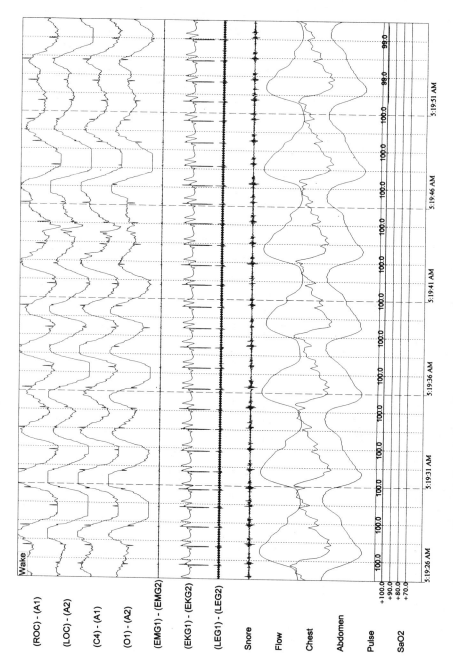

Figure 13. Typical effects of sweat artifact are shown in the EOG and EEG channels.

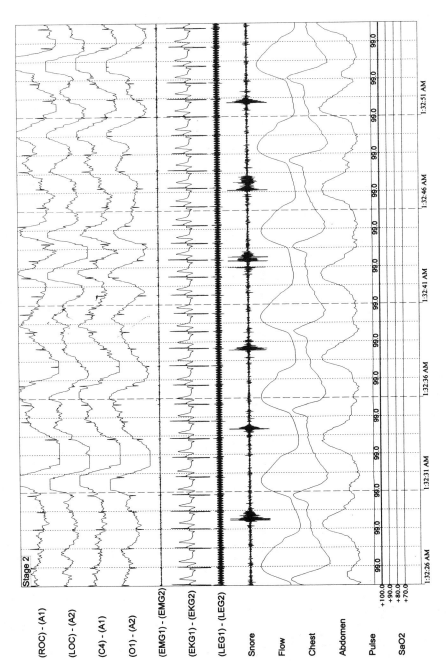

Figure 14. Typical respiratory artifact. Note that the waveforms are similar in the EOG, EEG, chest, abdomen, and nasal-oral airflow channels.

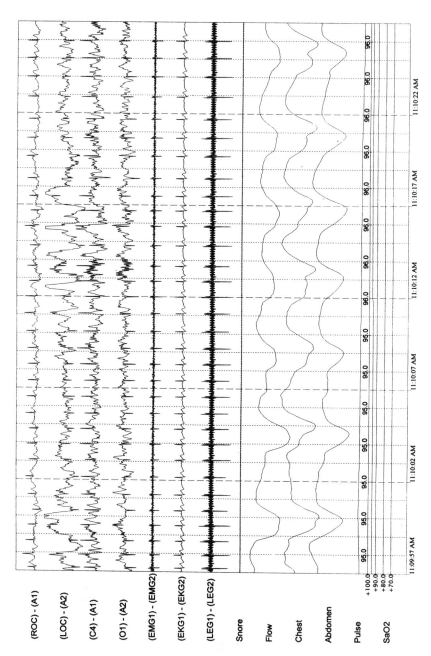

Figure 15. Typical EKG artifact. It is seen prominently in the EOG, EEG, EMG, and leg channels. This is a common occurrence but rarely affects accurate interpretation of the recording.

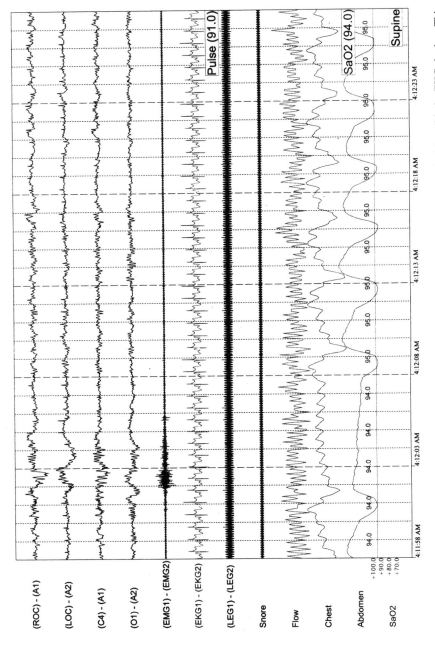

Figure 16. Ballistocardiogram or the effects of cardiac pulsations on the chest channel. Note that the waveform coincides with the EKG rhythm. This artifact may also be seen in the abdominal and/or airflow channel. Note additional artifact in flow channel.

7. OTHER DIAGNOSTIC TESTS IN SLEEP MEDICINE

Damien Stevens, MD

SLEEP DIARIES/SLEEP LOGS

1. What is a sleep diary or sleep log?

The main function of a sleep diary/sleep log is to document the total sleep time and bedtime/awake time. Many different forms exist with several different variations. Most include the time in bed, sleep onset time, awakening time, time awake during the night, and naps during the day. Some diaries include a scale of "mood" or energy level, and many include a space to document stressors, medications, caffeine or alcohol intake, and other factors that may affect sleep quality. Most diaries allow a 1- or 2-week collection period on each individual page. A sample sleep diary is shown in Figure 1.

2. When are sleep diaries or sleep logs indicated in the evaluation of patients?

They are useful for documenting several components of the sleep history. Obviously, sleep onset time can only be estimated since full polysomnography (PSG) is not performed and diaries are self-report only. Strengths of sleep diaries or sleep logs include the low cost and the fact they can be easily mailed. In addition, involving the patient in the diagnostic and treatment process can often be useful. Completion of a sleep diary prior to an office visit can especially be insightful into details of patients sleep.

3. How accurate are sleep diaries compared with actigraphy or polysomnography?

PSG has been compared with sleep diaries in at least one study evaluating narcoleptic and healthy control patients. The sleep-wake pattern by self-report was fairly accurate, but nap periods were underreported in the narcoleptic group. Actigraphy has also been shown to correlate with total sleep time estimates by sleep diaries/sleep logs in most studies. In patients with insomnia, however, sleep diaries were more significantly correlated than actigraphy with PSG total sleep time.

ACTIGRAPHY

4. Should sleep logs be recorded simultaneously with actigraphy?

Concomitant sleep diaries and actigraphy may allow a more accurate analysis of the sleep parameters. The sleep log provides additional information for defining artifacts and for determining bedtime and awake time.

5. What are indications for actigraphy in patients with a suspected sleep disorder?

This question is much debated, but a recent statement from the American Academy of Sleep Medicine states, "Actigraphy is not indicated for the routine diagnosis, assessment of severity, or management of any of the sleep disorders." This statement seems reasonable given the limitations of this method and the limited data in different sleep disorders. The statement later mentions two specific sleep disorders in which actigraphy may be useful. Insomnia may be assessed with actigraphy, along with treatment effects and any role of circadian rhythm disturbances, and actigraphy may assist in assessing the treatment response for restless legs syndrome (RLS) and periodic limb movement syndrome (PLMS).

		⇐ COMPLETE THIS SECTION AFTER GETTING OUT OF BED ⇒						⇐ COMPLETE AT END OF NEXT DAY ⇒		
Day & Date	Unusual stressors, time of alcohol & sleep medications	Time you went to bed	Time it took you to fall asleep	# of awakenings	*Amount of time awake	Time you got up for the day	Total sleep time	Sleepiness Rating (see below)	Fatigue Rating (see below)	Napping: time of day & sleep amount
Sunday 5/20/00	argument at dinner, 2 beers 6-8pm, Ambien 10 mg at 9:30pm	10pm	30 min	3	30 min	6am	7 hr	75	45	3pm 1 hr

* **Amount of time awake**: this is all the time you spent awake during the night, from the first time you awakened to the time you got out of bed. It does not include the time it took you to fall asleep initially.

SLEEPINESS AND FATIGUE RATING SCALE: (AVERAGE RATING FOR THE WHOLE DAY FOLLOWING A GIVEN SLEEP EPISODE)					
	0	25	50	75	...100
SLEEPINESS:	Extremely sleepy	Sleepy	Neither	Alert	Very alert
FATIGUE:	Extremely fatigued	Fatigued	Neither	Energetic	Very energetic

Figure 1. Sample sleep diary/sleep log includes sleepiness and fatigue ratings with notes regarding stressors, alcohol, or medications.

6. How does actigraphy work? How is it performed?

Actigraphy has been available for over 20 years; it works by using movement detectors or accelerometers. These instruments consist of a small, watch-size device that is usually placed on the wrist by an elastic band. A memory chip records these movements several times per second over days or weeks and stores the data. Computer programs are then used to analyze the data for activity/inactivity and sleep/wake parameters. Circadian data regarding amplitude of activity can also be reviewed. A sample actigraph result is shown in Figure 2.

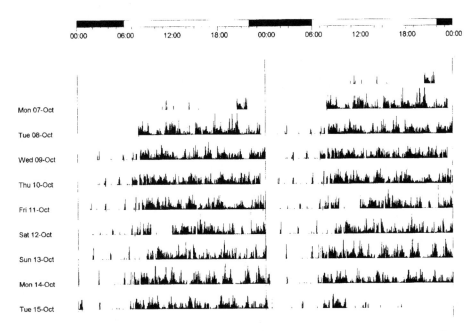

Figure 2. Sample actigraphy result from a healthy person with a sleep time from midnight to 8 AM. Note that each recorded line represents a 48-hour period, which overlaps with the preceding and following day.

7. How long should actigraphy be performed?

Actigraphy should usually be applied for at least three consecutive days. However, the length of time depends on why actigraphy is performed in the first place. Circadian disorders may require a more prolonged recording period.

8. Does it matter where the actigraph is placed?

There are conflicting data in regard to this question. Some studies have shown no difference in data collected from dominant wrist, nondominant wrist, ankle, or even trunk. Others studies have shown that wrist placement detects more movements than ankle or trunk placement. Dominant wrist may be better than nondominant wrist placement. In summary, the superiority of actigraphy placement on different body parts has not been established.

9. How accurate is actigraphy compared with polysomnography?

Actigraphy is highly correlated with PSG in differentiating sleep from wake, and the correlation with total sleep time is as high as 0.97. This high level of correlation has been found in adolescents and younger adults (20 to 30 years old), but in nursing home populations the correlation between actigraphy and PSG total sleep time was somewhat lower. Specific sleep parameters such as sleep onset may not be as accurate. In addition, actigraphy is less reliable in detecting sleep when the sleep is more frequently interrupted.

NOCTURNAL PENILE TUMESCENCE TESTING

10. How is nocturnal penile tumescence testing performed?

Nocturnal penile tumescence (NPT) or sleep-related erections (SREs) have been measured since the 1960s. Initially a mercury strain gage was used to measure penile circumference. Later a standardized scoring system with definitions of measurements and assessment of penile rigidity was added.

11. At what stage of sleep are SREs most commonly found?

The vast majority of SREs are temporally related to REM sleep. Typically, the erection initiates during the transition from NREM to REM sleep with full tumescence throughout REM. The penis then becomes flaccid again when NREM sleep commences.

12. How is penile rigidity measured?

Rigidity is defined as penile buckling resistance and is one of the most important components of the NPT test. Circumference usually correlates with rigidity, but dissociation between the two measurements may occur. To measure rigidity, a patient is awakened during a SRE and the technician applies a force parallel to the shaft of the penis. The force is progressively increased until buckling of the penis is noted.

13. What is the role of nocturnal penile tumescence testing?

The main goals are to record penile rigidity during maximal erection and to obtain a calibrated penile circumference measurement throughout the recording. NPT testing was initially developed to differentiate "organic" from psychogenic or behavioral causes of impotence. It is assumed that the presence of "normal" nocturnal erections excludes the possibility of anatomic causes of impotence such as insufficient blood flow. However, neurologic deficits and androgen deficiency are known to cause impotence despite normal NPT test results. In addition, mixed "organic" and psychogenic causes certainly coexist in some patients so that a clear distinction between the two causes may not be possible.

14. What is the normal finding on NPT testing?

Several large studies done in several age groups have been published. In summary, SREs are found with high consistency in all groups of healthy men with an average of 3 to 4 episodes per night. In terms of rigidity, the average minimum force required for intercourse ranges from 500 to 650 gm.

CEPHALOMETRICS

15. What is cephalometry?

Cephalometry is a plain lateral radiograph of the head and neck. It is used to examine the upper airway and craniofacial structures. The head must be stabilized during the radiograph exposure, and the radiograph should be obtained after complete expiration to ensure standardization.

16. What is the role of cephalometrics in evaluating a patient suspected of having sleep-disordered breathing?

Cephalometrics may be useful in evaluating patients with retronagthia and/or micronagthia. Some sleep specialists also find cephalometrics useful in evaluating the efficacy of oral appliances or when upper airway surgery is considered.

17. What measurements are made during cephalometrics?

Several different measurements are made during cephalometrics. Patients with sleep apnea have smaller retroposed mandibles, narrow posterior airway space, enlarged tongue and soft palate, inferiorly positioned hyoid bones, and reposition of the maxilla compared with healthy controls. Specific measurements often reported include the maxilla to cranial base, mandible to cranial base, posterior airway space, soft palate length, and distance of hyoid from inferior mandible. Figure 3 shows these measurements.

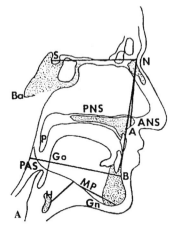

Figure 3. Cephalometric measurements used to evaluate patients for SAHS. SNA = maxilla to cranial base; SNB = mandible to cranial base; PAS = posterior airway space; PNS = length of soft palate; MP-H = distance of hyoid from inferior mandible. (From Lee-Chiong TL, Sateia M, Carskadon MA. Sleep Medicine. Philadelphia, Hanley & Belfus, 2002, with permission.)

18. How accurate are cephalometrics for sleep apnea hyopnea syndrome (SAHS)?
Only one variable, mandibular body length, has consistently been shown to differentiate patients with SAHS from healthy controls. Therefore, cephalometrics are not a very useful diagnostic tool for SAHS.

19. Are cephalometrics cost-effective?
No study has reported the cost-effectiveness of cephalometrics. Even though the test is widely available, easily performed, and relatively inexpensive compared with other radiographic tests, it is unlikely cephalometric tests are cost-effective due to the minimal additional information that they provide.

PORTABLE SLEEP STUDIES AND NOCTURNAL OXIMETRY

20. What are the different types of sleep recordings?
Sleep recordings range from level I to level IV, depending on the number of parameters recorded and other data analyzed. The table below shows the criteria for these different levels.

Sleep Recording Categories (Six-hour Recording Minimum)

	Level I: Standard PSG	Level II: Comprehensive Portable PSG	Level III: Modified Portable Sleep Apnea Testing	Level IV: Continuous Single or Dual Bioparameter Recording
Parameters	Minimum of 7, including EEG, EOG, chin EMG, ECG, airflow, respiratory effort, oxygen saturation	Minimum of 7, including EEG, EOG, chin EMG, ECG or heart rate, airflow, respiratory effort, oxygen saturation	Minimum of 4, including ventilation (at least 2 channels of respiratory movement, or respiratory movement and airflow), heart rate or ECG, oxygen saturation	Minimum of 1

Table continued on next page

Sleep Recording Categories (Six-hour Recording Minimum) (Cont.)

	Level I: Standard PSG	Level II: Comprehensive Portable PSG	Level III: Modified Portable Sleep Apnea Testing	Level IV: Continuous Single or Dual Bioparameter Recording
Body position	Documented or measured	May be objectively measured	May be objectively measured	Not measured
Leg movement	EMG or motion sensor desirable but optional	EMG or motion sensor desirable but optional	May be recorded	Not recorded
Personnel	In constant attendance	Not in attendance	Not in attendance	Not in attendance
Interventions	Possible	Not possible	Not possible	Not possible

PSG = polysomnography, EEG = electroencephalogram, EOG = electrooculogram, EMG = electromyogram, ECG = electrocardiogram.

21. When are unattended portable sleep recordings an acceptable alternative to laboratory polysomnography?

In 1994 the American Sleep Disorders Association (ASDA) Standards of Practice Committee stated there portable sleep recording has a limited role. The limited indications included (1) patients with severe clinical symptoms of SAHS needing urgent treatment, (2) patients incapable of undergoing laboratory polysomnography, and (3) follow-up studies to evaluate response to therapy. In an updated statement in 1997, the ASDA stated that type 3 studies might be appropriate in patients with a high index of suspicion for SAHS but added that negative studies should be followed by laboratory polysomnography.

22. What are the advantages and limitations of portable sleep recordings?

Advantages include accessibility, convenience, patient acceptability, a familiar sleep environment, and cost savings. The main limitation is that the lack of a technician may lead to inadequate data due to artifacts, lost leads, and inability to titrate continuous positive airway pressure (CPAP), if needed. Studies have shown an at-home failure rate of 10% to 20%. Technicians are also unavailable to intervene for CPAP mask intolerance, request different sleep positions, or add supplemental oxygen, if needed.

23. How cost-effective are portable sleep recordings?

Too few data are available to answer this question adequately. Simpler recordings, level III or IV, cost less, but if verification of a sleep disorder is required or if there is a high rate of data loss or insufficient recording, this cost savings may not be realized. Diagnosis of SAHS also requires an additional night for titration of CPAP therapy unless an autotitrating positive airway pressure device is used. The common use of "split night" studies avoids a second PSG night in some patients.

24. Is overnight oximetry an adequate screening test for SAHS?

Oximetry alone has been evaluated in several large studies. In most studies a negative test is usually useful for ruling out sleep apnea, but a positive test requires further confirmatory testing. Combining snoring with oximetry increases specificity but has little effect on sensitivity.

25. How useful is nasal pressure measurement in the diagnosis of SAHS?

Nasal pressure transducers have been shown to have a high sensitivity (from 97% to 100%) with a lower specificity, when using esophageal pressure monitoring as a gold standard.

BIBLIOGRAPHY

1. American Sleep Disorders Association: Practice parameters for the use of actigraphy in the clinical assessment of sleep disorders: An American Sleep Disorders Association Report. Sleep 18(4): 285–287, 1995.
2. Boehlecke B: Controversies in monitoring and testing for sleep-disordered breathing. Curr Opin Pulmon Med 7(6):372–380, 2001.
3. Ferber R, Millman R, Coppola M, et al: Portable recording in the assessment of obstructive sleep apnea: ASDA Standards of Practice. Sleep 17:378–392, 1994.
4. Lee-Chiong TL, Sateia M, Carskadon MA (eds): Sleep Medicine. Philadelphia, Hanley & Belfus, 2002.
5. Sadeh A, Acebo C: The role of actigraphy in sleep medicine. Sleep Med Rev 6:113–124, 2002.
6. Sadeh A, Hauri PJ, Kripke DF, Lavie P: The role of actigraphy in the evaluation of sleep disorders: An American Sleep Disorders Association Review. Sleep 18(4):288–302, 1995.
7. Standards Practice Committee of the American Sleep Disorders Association: Practice parameters for the use of portable recording in the assessment of obstructive sleep apnea: ASDA Standards of Practice. Sleep 17:372–377, 1994.

II. Specific Sleep Disorders

8. SLEEP APNEA-HYPOPNEA SYNDROME AND PRIMARY SNORING

Damien Stevens, MD

SLEEP APNEA-HYPOPNEA SYNDROME

Epidemiology

1. How common is sleep apnea-hypopnea syndrome or obstructive sleep apnea?

The answer depends on the definition of sleep apnea-hypopnea syndrome (SAHS). Using an apnea-hypopnea index of 5 or greater, the prevalence is 9% for females and 24% for males. If the patient is symptomatic with an apnea-hypopnea index of 5 or greater, the numbers are 2% for females and 4% for males. Different studies have found a wide variability in prevalence but almost all find that at least 1% of their population, male and female, have symptomatic SAHS.

2. How does the prevalence of obstructive sleep apnea vary with gender and race?

Males have a higher prevalence compared with females. Certain races are more prone to sleep apnea based on epidemiologic studies. For instance, African-Americans have a higher prevalence of SAHS compared with other ethnic groups. The Asian population is also thought to be at higher risk, even with a normal body mass index (BMI). (*Note:* BMI is determined by dividing weight in kilograms by height in meters squared). This finding is thought to be due to craniofacial differences, such as retrognathia.

3. What are the most common risk factors for SAHS?

The common risk factors for SAHS include obesity, male gender, postmenopausal status, craniofacial abnormalities, and abnormal upper airway anatomy (i.e., macroglossia or enlarged tonsils). Nearly all measures of obesity (BMI, waist circumference, and waist-to-hip ratio) predict the presence of SAHS. Comorbid conditions such as cardiac or pulmonary disease may also predispose patients to SAHS. Familial factors play some role through genetic inheritance. Finally, environmental factors such as alcohol, smoking, and sedative/hypnotics can produce or worsen SAHS.

4. Do risk factors for SAHS vary with age?

Risk factors vary with age to some degree, mainly for pediatric patients. One of the major differences is enlarged tonsils, which increase the odds of SAHS much greater in children than in adults. Male gender and obesity appear to increase the risk of SAHS in adults but not in pediatric patients. On the other hand, genetic inheritance seems to play a more significant role in pediatric patients than in adults. Although not a risk factor, daytime sleepiness is typically milder or even nonexistent in pediatric patients in contrast to adult patients.

Pathophysiology

5. What is the basic determinant of upper airway collapse in SAHS patients?

The pharynx is a collapsible tube that is acted upon by intraluminal and extraluminal pressure, thereby producing a transmural pressure. The extraluminal forces are due to the surrounding tissue and tend to collapse the upper airway, whereas the intraluminal pressure is reduced in patients with a narrowed upper airway. Airway obstruction occurs if the dilating forces are exceeded by the collapsing forces.

6. What is the role of upper airway crowding in SAHS?

Upper airway crowding leads to a narrowed upper airway. The resultant decrease in cross-sectional area of the airway, then leads to a reduction in the intraluminal pressure. When intraluminal pressure is exceeded by extraluminal pressure, airway collapse occurs.

7. What is the role of the neurologic system in SAHS?

Pharyngeal dilator muscles surprisingly have increased activity in patients with SAHS compared with controls, but this increased activity is diminished after sleep onset. This decrease after sleep onset at least partially contributes to upper airway collapse. Neuromuscular stimulation applied intraorally may improve upper airway patency by directly increasing muscle tone of the upper airway. The genioglossus muscle appears to play a major role as well as the soft palate muscles (levator veli palatini, tensor veli palatini, palatoglossus, palatopharyngeus, and superior pharyngeal constrictor muscles). Hypoglossal nerve stimulation has been used in patients with SAHS with some increase in inspiratory airflow, but research is still ongoing.

8. What role does gravity play in SAHS?

The role of gravity is suggested by several clinical finding in SAHS. Gravity probably plays a role in the "positionality" of SAHS or the worsening of airway narrowing in the supine vs. the lateral position. The National Aeronautics and Space Administration (NASA) completed a study of astronauts while they were in orbit (no gravity) and found an improvement in the AHI compared with sleep on earth. However, because none of the subjects had significant sleep apnea, the effect of no gravity has not been evaluated in patients with SAHS.

9. What have imaging studies of the upper airway shown in patients with SAHS?

Several different methods of upper airway imaging have been used. The simplest of these methods is cephalometrics, which is essentially a lateral skull plain radiograph. Several studies have shown a strong correlation between certain cephalometric measures and the presence of SAHS. More recently, computed tomographic scanning and magnetic resonance imaging have been used to assess upper airway patency during the awake and sleep states. These studies led to the discovery that patients with SAHS have narrowing in the lateral dimension of their airway, whereas the anteroposterior distance was essentially normal. In other words, the long axis of the elliptical airway was oriented in the coronal plane for normal subjects and in the sagittal plane for patients with SAHS.

10. How do apneas and hypopneas differ?

According to the position paper of the American Academy of Sleep Medicine (AASM), an **apnea** is scored when nasal-oral airflow is less than 20% compared with the baseline for at least 10 seconds. An obstructive apnea also requires evidence of continued respiratory effort, as measured by abdominal and/or thoracic monitoring.

Hypopneas are typically defined as a 20-80% decrement in nasal-oral airflow compared with the baseline. Hypopneas must be also accompanied by either a 4% oxyhemoglobin desaturation or an electroencephalographic (EEG) arousal, depending on which specific definition is used. An example of an obstructive apnea is shown in Figure 1, and a hypopnea is shown in Figure 2.

11. How does the physiology of a mixed apnea differ from the physiology of other apneas?

Mixed apneas typically begin as a central apnea with no evidence of effort or airflow. Then a resumption of effort ensues during the apneic period, but no airflow is produced. Occasionally the obstructive component may precede the central apnea.

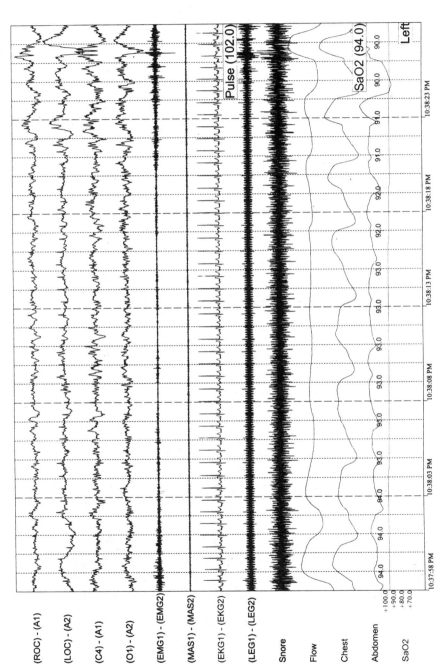

Figure 1. Obstructive apnea. Continued respiratory effort is seen with deflection of the abdominal and thoracic channels but absence of nasal-oral airflow.

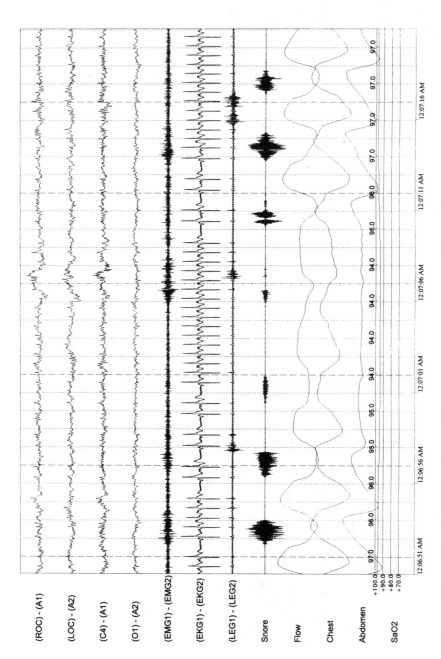

Figure 2. Hypopnea. Decreased nasal-oral airflow is seen without complete absence of flow. Oxygen desaturation due to a previous hypopnea is recorded with the typical delay in desaturation after an episode of hypopnea.

Classification

12. Are apneas and hypopneas classified separately?
Typically hypopneas and apneas are summed together to obtain an apnea-hypopnea index (AHI), also known as respiratory disturbance index (RDI). The AHI reflects the average number of hypopneas and apneas during recorded sleep. It is thought that the consequences of an apnea and hypopnea are similar, even though the physiology may be different. In the pediatric population, however, apneas are considered more significant than hypopneas.

13. How is the severity of SAHS classified?
The classification of severity of SAHS is the average number of hypopneas and apneas per hour of sleep (AHI or RDI). As of this writing, the proposed classification by the Sleep Medicine Task Force is as follows:

AHI	Classification of Severity
≤ 5	Normal
5-15	Mild obstructive sleep apnea
5-30	Moderate obstructive sleep apnea
> 30	Severe obstructive sleep apnea

14. How is oxygen desaturation classified?
Oxygen desaturation is not included in the classification scheme of the Sleep Medicine Task Force, but some sleep specialists include a marker of its severity, such as **lowest oxygen saturation** or **oxygen desaturation index**. The oxygen saturation index is typically defined as the percent of the total sleep time during which the patient had an oxygen saturation below a designated level (often 90%). The severity of daytime sleepiness may also be assessed and classified as mild, moderate, or severe, depending on whether the desaturations produce minor, moderate, or marked daytime impairment.

15. What does the term *positional apnea* mean?
Some patients may present with apnea mainly during sleep in the supine position. The prevalence of this disorder remains unknown as well as the exact definition that should be used. Many specialists simply require that the majority of the respiratory events occur while the patient is supine, but a more precise definition should be an elevated AHI in the supine position with a normal AHI when the patient is not in the supine position. This distinction is relevant in deciding treatment, because a patient with an elevated AHI in the nonsupine position may require different treatment from a patient with positional apnea.

Diagnosis

16. What is the gold standard for diagnosis of SAHS?
A polysomnogram is considered the gold standard. The number of channels monitored may differ among sleep laboratories, but the essential components include oximetry, a measure of respiratory effort, nasal-oral airflow measurement, and EEG monitoring. A study period resembling the patient's typical sleep period is considered ideal, but a "daytime" study can also be used to diagnose SAHS. Continuous oximetry may also suggest SAHS, but there are other causes than SAHS for nocturnal hypoxemia. Newer positive airway pressure (PAP) units, called auto-PAP, can detect either airflow limitation or snoring as an indicator of SAHS. They appear to be fairly accurate, but their exact role in the diagnosis and management of patients with SAHS remains undefined.

17. What are common symptoms in patients with SAHS?
The most common symptom in most studies is snoring. Other common complaints are snorting, choking, gasping, stopped breathing, morning headaches, impotence, nocturia (nocturnal uri-

nation), and daytime sleepiness. Occasionally patients report fatigue rather than sleepiness, impaired intellectual performance, and even mood or behavioral complaints. In children, hyperactivity and poor school performance are commonly noted.

18. Discuss the sensitivity and specificity of these symptoms.

Snoring alone has a sensitivity of 71% but a specificity of only 32%. Snoring with apneas has a sensitivity of 23% but a specificity of 94%. Combining other symptoms with physical examination findings increases both the sensitivity and specificity, but the maximal value probably remains below 90%.

19. What is the role of esophageal manometry in diagnosing sleep-disordered breathing?

Esophageal manometry using an esophageal balloon is the only practical way to assess pleural pressure in the sleep laboratory. Pleural pressure is important because it reflects respiratory effort, and the syndrome of "upper airway resistance" is thought to be due to progressive increases in respiratory effort. For many patients with straightforward SAHS, this differentiation is not critical, but in patients with snoring and repeated arousals due to progressive upper airway narrowing or respiratory effort-related arousals (RERAs), this diagnosis may be missed. On the other hand, an esophageal balloon involves some minor risks and can affect sleep architecture; furthermore, the true existence of "upper airway resistance syndrome" is still debated. In addition, nasal pressure transducers through a nasal cannula have become available recently that are fairly accurate and may negate the need for esophageal balloon manometry.

Prognosis and Treatment

20. Describe the natural history of untreated SAHS.

Few studies have attempted to answer this question, but before the introduction of continuous positive airway pressure (CPAP), therapy some studies followed patients who received "conservative" therapy. Conservative treatment typically consisted of weight loss and occasionally upper airway surgery with only mild benefit. A mortality rate of 6% per 5-8 years has been quoted, but coexistent medical disorders were not reported in detail. Studies in elderly populations have often found no relationship between SAHS and increased mortality. Mild SAHS often evolves into more severe sleep apnea over time. Occasionally SAHS becomes less severe but rarely ever disappears.

21. What are the main types of treatment options for SAHS?

CPAP has become the gold standard for treatment of SAHS. Other options include weight loss, surgical therapy, pharmacologic agents, positional therapy, and oral appliances.

22. What was the first surgical treatment for obstructive sleep apnea?

The first surgical treatment was tracheostomy. It was known for several years that tracheostomy bypassed the upper airway, thereby avoiding apneic episodes. In the 1960s, Ikematsu of Japan and in the 1980s Fujita of the United States reported surgery of the upper airway directed at the treatment of snoring. Fujita's work eventually led to the procedure known as uvulo-palatopharyngoplasty (UPPP)).

23. What different pharmacologic agents have been used for SAHS? How effective are they?

Several different agents have been used with limited success. Protriptyline has been shown to modestly reduce the AHI but rarely cures SAHS. It may have a role in REM-related SAHS specifically. Progesterone has little effect except in the setting of obesity-hypoventilation syndrome. Seritonergic agents have been studied in animal models with good results, especially in bulldogs. But to date they appear to have a minimal effect in humans. Acetazolamide may reduce the AHI, but few studies have been performed and side effects limits its usefulness. Theophylline, nicotine, and thyroid supplements have been studied but show no significant effect.

24. How effective is weight loss for SAHS?

Weight loss can be highly effective for the treatment of SAHS, but consistent prolonged weight loss is extremely difficult to achieve. Some patients redevelop SAHS even if weight loss is maintained. The amount of weight loss required to improve or resolve SAHS varies greatly among different patients. In the most scientifically sound study, which was conducted over a 5 month period in 15 participants, a mean weight loss of 9.6 kg was obtained with a pre-weight loss AHI of 55 and a post-weight loss AHI of 29.2. Bariatric surgery to induce weight loss appears to be the most consistently successful method to achieve weight loss and improve or even cure SAHS, but double-blind, placebo controlled studies are lacking.

25. When was continuous positive airway pressure first developed?

The use of CPAP was first reported in 1981 by Sullivan and Issa in Australia.

26. How does continuous positive airway pressure prevent apneas?

The application of CPAP prevents upper airway collapse, thereby preventing apneas. The airway pressure counteracts the collapsing force found in patients with SAHS. The term *pneumatic splint* is often used to describe these physiologic effects.

27. What are the physiologic effects of CPAP?

CPAP physiologically resembles positive end-expiratory pressure (PEEP). It increases intrathoracic pressure and therefore can have several physiologic effects. At higher levels CPAP may decrease preload by decreasing venous return. It has the potential to induce hypotension with decreased cardiac output. This effect is rare in most outpatients, probably because they are euvolemic and hemodynamically stable.

28. How effective is CPAP for the treatment of SAHS?

CPAP is almost completely effective in the alleviation of obstructive apneas and hypopneas as long as the patient tolerates the treatment. Some patients may still have persistently low oxygen saturation levels despite correction of SAHS, which often implies underlying cardiac, pulmonary, or neuromuscular disease.

29. How is compliance with CPAP assessed?

Initially patients were simply asked how often and how long they used the CPAP unit. Eventually hour meters, which record the time during which the CPAP units were turned on, were installed, and it was found that patient reports are highly inaccurate compared with "time-on" readings from CPAP units. Patients consistently overestimated CPAP usage. Later, compliance monitors that monitored time at effective pressure rather than time the units were turned on showed that often patients were turning on the CPAP units without actually using them.

30. How compliant are patients with CPAP?

Studies report a wide variation in compliance rates, and the definition of compliance also varies greatly. Most studies have reported a mean CPAP usage between 4.7 and 5.1 hours nightly. Many researchers now use 4 hours as the minimum time needed to designate compliance since it appears that this minimum is required for adequate daytime performance. Of interest, some studies have found that long-term compliance can be predicted by the compliance rate after 1 week of CPAP therapy in the majority of patients.

31. How can CPAP compliance be increased?

Many studies have attempted to increase CPAP compliance through a multitude of methods. Cognitive behavioral therapy, a "compliance clinic," a desensitization program, and other methods have not consistently been shown to increase compliance rates. Bilevel positive airway pressure (BiPAP) may be useful in some intolerant patients, but randomized studies have shown long-term CPAP and BiPAP compliance rates to be the same.

32. What factors predict CPAP compliance?
No factors have consistently predicted CPAP compliance rates. The severity of SAHS as measured by desaturation or AHI are poor predictors, and no other polysomnographic markers have been found. Patient's perception of benefit from CPAP appears to be the only useful predictor.

33. When is bilevel positive airway pressure indicated for SAHS?
The vast majority of patients with SAHS are adequately treated with CPAP therapy. BiPAP has the potential benefit of a lower expiratory airway pressure since the "bilevel" capabilities of the device allow an inspiratory and expiratory setting that can be adjusted separately. Many clinicians believe that this lower expiratory pressure may increase patient comfort and therefore tolerance of BiPAP compared with CPAP therapy. However, too low an expiratory pressure setting may induce continued airway collapse so that SAHS may not be adequately treated. In addition, although theoretically BiPAP may lead to increased compliance compared with CPAP, studies that investigated this possibility have not found it to be true.

34. What surgical options are available for correction of SAHS?
Several different surgical options are available for the treatment of SAHS. The first treatment directed at SAHS was tracheotomy. This procedure bypassed the upper airway, thereby alleviating upper airway obstruction. Since then several different surgical approaches have been developed, along with different combinations of surgical interventions. The table below lists specific procedures. Tonsillectomy in the pediatric population is often curative, whereas in adults it usually has minimal effect on SAHS.

Surgical Procedures for SAHS and Primary Snoring

Tracheotomy
Uvulopalatopharyngoplasty
Genioglossal advancement
Genioglossal advancement with hyoid myotomy
Tonsillectomy
Maxillomandibular osteotomy and advancement
Lingualplasty/laser midline glossectomy

35. What is the role of uvulopalatopharyngoplasty for therapy of SAHS?
Some sleep specialist believe that UPPP has no role in patients with significant sleep-disordered breathing, but others consider it a treatment option if patients are unable to tolerate CPAP therapy. There is little likelihood that moderate or severe SAHS will be sufficiently treated with UPPP alone, but an occasional patient experiences significant benefit. The ability to predict which patients are most likely to respond to UPPP is critically important, but this question remains unanswered.

36. What types of oral appliances are used for the treatment of SAHS?
The two main types are tongue repositioning devices and mandibular repositioning devices. Several different types of both devices are available.

37. How are oral appliances thought to work?
Both types of devices are thought to increase upper airway patency by decreasing collapsibility.

38. How effective are oral appliances for SAHS?
Study results vary widely due to the difference in devices, different baseline severity of SAHS, and different definitions of "success." To summarize several studies, 54–81% of patients have a reduction in the AHI by 50%, and 51–64% have an AHI less than 10 while using an oral appliance. Overall, the more severe the SAHS, the less likely it is that oral appliances will be curative.

39. Are there any predictors of oral appliance efficacy?

Predictors of efficacy include younger age, lower BMI, positional SAHS, and increased protrusion with the appliance. Patients with craniofacial abnormalities predisposing to upper airway narrowing may also benefit more from oral appliances.

40. What are the most common side effects of oral appliances?

Temporomandibular joint pain appears to be the most serious adverse effect, but in most patients it resolves with cessation of oral appliance use. Altered occlusion, dry mouth, tooth discomfort, excessive salivation, and jaw pain are also reported. Occasionally, SAHS may be worsened by oral appliances through an unknown mechanism.

41. What new technology is available to diagnose and treat SAHS?

As mentioned previously, newer diagnostic and treatment units for SAHS have been produced in the past few years. These autotitrating devices may use a microphone for snoring and have the ability to detect airflow limitation, suggestive of SAHS. Airflow limitation occurs when increasing the airway pressure does not lead to increased flow through the airway, indicating a collapsed airway. More recently, some systems use peripheral arterial tonometry as an indirect indicator of apneic events.

PRIMARY SNORING

42. How common is snoring?

The published rates vary widely, depending on several factors. The presence of a bed partner typically doubles the reported rate of snoring. In addition, how often the snoring occurs, how the poll was conducted (by phone, mail, face-to-face interview), and the country where the study was completed affect the prevalence rate. The prevalence ranges from 5% to 86%, with a mean of 32%, in men and from 2% to 57%, with a mean of 21%, in women.

43. How is snoring measured, subjectively and objectively?

To date, there is still no agreed upon standard subjective or objective measure for snoring, but several different measures can be used. Subjective measures of snoring simply use self-report or a bed partner's report as to whether snoring is present. The bed partner is obviously better qualified to report whether a person snores. However, because observers have different arousal thresholds and tolerance of nocturnal disruptions, they may differ greatly when they report the frequency and loudness of the snoring. Objective measures usually include a microphone recording, but the distance from the patient to the microphone varies greatly among different studies, and no "standard" decibel level is used to define snoring.

44. What causes snoring?

Snoring is caused by vibration of the soft tissues of the pharynx, soft palate, and sometimes even the uvula. It usually occurs during inspiration and expiration. The snoring sound may vary, depending on whether the person is using nasal, oral, or oronasal breathing.

45. What are the risk factors for snoring?

Obesity is the most common risk factor, but male gender and family history are also important.

46. What are the treatment options for snoring?

Avoidance of agents that worsen snoring, such as alcohol, smoking, muscle-relaxing agents, and sleep deprivation, is the first step. Weight loss, oral appliances, upper airway surgery, and position training may be useful. In rare cases, CPAP may also be used.

47. What is the role of nasal dilators for snoring?

The majority of nasal dilators have either not been studied or were poorly studied. For the most part, they are only moderately useful. But at least they are usually inexpensive.

48. Does snoring cause daytime sleepiness?

By definition, primary snoring represents only snoring without arousals or daytime sleepiness. However, some use the term "upper airway resistance syndrome" to designate patients who have snoring as a sign of increased upper airway resistance, which then leads to arousals and secondary daytime sleepiness.

49. What are the health consequences of snoring?

There still is a significant amount of debate about the health consequences of snoring. Several studies have shown an association between snoring and hypertension, but this association has not been found in all studies, and obesity is a confounding factor because it is common in both diseases. An association with cerebrovascular disease and coronary artery disease has also been reported, but these data are less convincing.

BIBLIOGRAPHY

1. Ayappa I, Rapoport DM: The upper airway in sleep: Physiology of the pharynx. Sleep Med Rev 7:9-33, 2003.
2. Fairbanks DNF, Mickelson SA, Woodson BT: Snoring and Obstructive Sleep Apnea, 3rd ed. Philadelphia, Lippincott Williams & Wilkins, 2003.
3. Ferguson KA: The role of oral appliance therapy in the treatment of obstructive sleep apnea. Clin Chest Med 24:355-364, 2003.
4. Flemons WW: Clinical practice: Obstructive sleep apnea. N Engl J Med 347:498-504, 2002.
5. Hoffstein V: Snoring, Chest 109:201-222, 1996.
6. Ivanhoe JR, Attanasio R: Sleep disorders and oral devices. Dent Clin North Am 45:733-758, 2001.
7. Lee-Chiong T, Mohsenin V: Sleep-related breathing disorders: New developments. Clin Chest Med 24:2, 2003.
8. Li KK: Surgical management of obstructive sleep apnea. Clin Chest Med 24:365-370, 2003.
9. Littner M, Hirshkowitz M, Davila D, et al: Practice parameters for the use of auto-titrating continuous positive airway pressure devices for titrating pressures and treating adult patients with obstructive sleep apnea syndrome. An American Academy of Sleep Medicine report. Sleep 25:143-147, 2002.
10. Meyer TK, Woodson T: Surgical management of snoring and obstructive sleep apnea. West Med J 102:28-31, 2003.
11. Sateia MJ: Neuropsychological impairment and quality of life in obstructive sleep apnea Clin Chest Med 24:249-259, 2003.
12. Smith I, Lasserson T, Wright J: Drug treatments for obstructive sleep apnoea. Cochrane Database Syst Rev (2):CD003002, 2002.

9. CENTRAL SLEEP APNEA

Damien Stevens, MD

EPIDEMIOLOGY

1. When was central sleep apnea first described?

Gastaut and his collaborators first described central sleep apnea (CSA) in 1966. They defined central apneas as an absence of airflow and respiratory effort lasting at least 10 seconds.

2. How common is central sleep apnea?

No large epidemiologic survey has been conducted to answer this question. All agree that CSA is much less common than obstructive sleep apnea. Some sleep centers report that predominantly central apneas are found in only about 10% of all their patients with sleep-disordered breathing.

3. What is the most common disease process causing central sleep apnea?

Although no epidemiologic study has evaluated this question, congestive heart failure is probably the most common cause of CSA.

4. With what type of sleep-disordered breathing should a patient be diagnosed when both central and obstructive apneas are present?

No consensus or guidelines address this question. If a significant number of hypopneas and obstructive apneas are present, continuous positive airway pressure (CPAP) therapy is indicated. Often the central apneas decrease or resolve with CPAP.

5. How many apneas should be present before central apnea is diagnosed?

Once again, no studies have been published detailing a normal central apnea index. Most sleep specialists consider less than 5 central apneas per hour normal, but more important than the index is the possibility of associated comorbid disease.

6. Are central apneas ever "benign"?

"Post-arousal" central apneas are commonly seen in patients without significant sleep or daytime complaints. There is no agreement on how frequent these apneas must be to be considered "pathologic."

PATHOPHYSIOLOGY

7. What factors lead to post-arousal central apneas?

Several physiologic phenomena may play a role in this process. The acute awakening changes the carbon dioxide response threshold. Acute hyperventilation at the time of arousal may also decrease the arterial carbon dioxide level enough to cause a central apnea.

8. Describe the physiologic basis of central apneas and periodic breathing due to altitude.

At high altitude, the ambient oxygen pressure is lower, thereby leading to hyperventilation. This hyperventilation leads to hypocapnia, which then leads to "ventilatory instability." This "instability" describes the periodic episodes of hyperpnea and apnea, which cause an "overshooting," then an "undershooting" of the ventilatory response.

CLASSIFICATION

9. What is the most common classification system for central sleep apnea syndrome? What are the two broad catergories?

Many sleep specialists classify patients with sleep apnea by whether the carbon dioxide level is elevated or normal as hypercapnic or nonhypercapnic CSA syndrome, respectively. The most common causes of CSA with normal daytime carbon dioxide or eucapnia is probably Cheyne-Stokes respiration. Elevated carbon dioxide levels or hypercapnia is found in patients with central alveolar hypoventilation syndrome, which is usually idiopathic. Others classify CSA as either primary or secondary, depending on whether the patient has a predisposing factor.

10. What does the term *periodic breathing* mean?

Periodic breathing describes a certain abnormal breathing pattern. There are several components to this type of breathing. Tachypnea (faster breathing rate) alternating with bradypnea (slower breathing rate) is noted as well as periods of hyperpnea (deeper breathing) alternating with apnea (absent breathing). The terms *crescendo* and *decrescendo* breathing are also used to describe this pattern. Periodic breathing is evident when the depth of the tidal volume is graphed against time. Figure 1 shows the breathing pattern as recorded on polysomnography.

11. Describe the relationship among central sleep apnea, periodic breathing, and Cheyne-Stokes respiration.

CSA simply means sleep interrupted by central apneas. Periodic breathing, as mentioned above, denotes periods of hyperpnea and tachypnea alternating with hypopnea and bradypnea. Some sleep specialists differentiate periodic breathing from Cheyne-Stokes respiration based on whether a central apnea is present and classify patients with intervening central apneas rather than hypopnea/bradypnea as having Cheyne-Stokes respiration with central sleep apnea (CSR-CSA). Therefore, Cheyne-Stokes respiration may be viewed as a subtype of central sleep apnea (Figs. 2 and 3).

12. What risk factors and disease processes that lead to central sleep apnea?
Cardiac disorders
  • Heart failure
  • Valvular dysfunction
Neurologic disorders
  • Stroke
  • Congenital malformations
  • Infection
  • Malignancies
  • Neuromuscular
  • Neurodegenerative diseases
  • Cervical cordotomy
Medications
Altitude
Pregnancy

DIAGNOSIS

13. What is the gold standard diagnostic test for central sleep apnea?

Standard polysomnography is the gold standard diagnostic procedure. Accurate measurement of respiratory effort is essential to make this diagnosis since absence of effort is consistent with a central apnea, whereas persistent effort without airflow occurs during obstructive apneas. Figure 4 shows how a central apnea appears on a standard polysomnography. If respiratory effort is present but not measured, the event will inappropriately be labeled a central apnea. This is

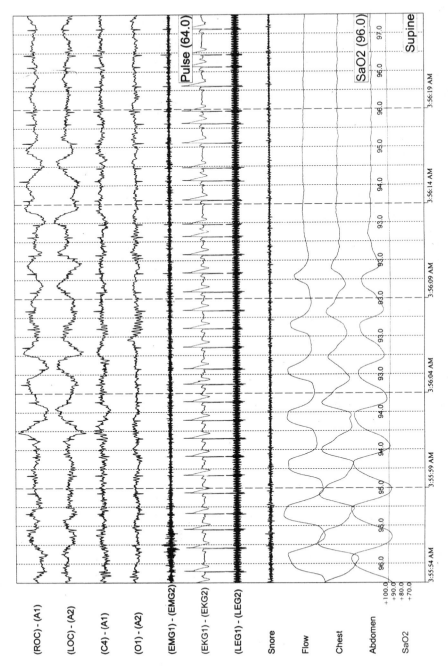

Figure 1. Cheyne-Stokes respiration. Note the waxing/waning or crescendo/decrescendo breathing pattern with an intervening apnea during a 30-second epoch.

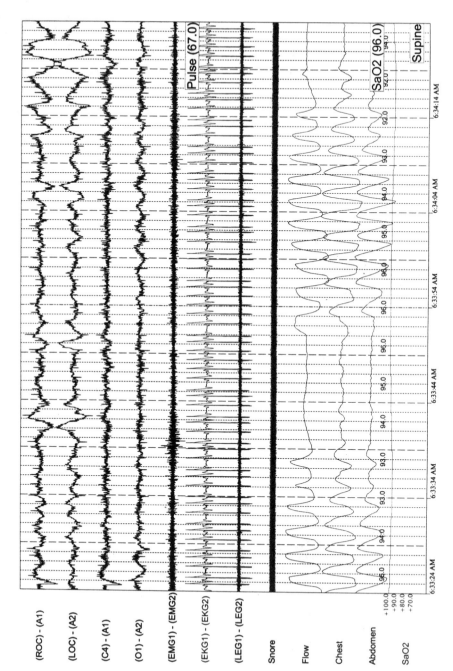

Figure 2. Cheyne-Stokes respiration. The breathing pattern may be even more evident with the timeline changed to 60-second epoch.

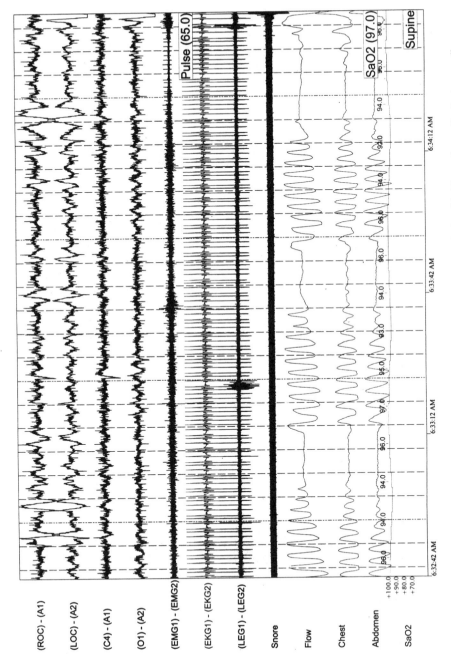

Figure 3. Cheyne-Stokes respiration. This figure shows the same breathing event depicted in Figure 2 on a 2-minute recording.

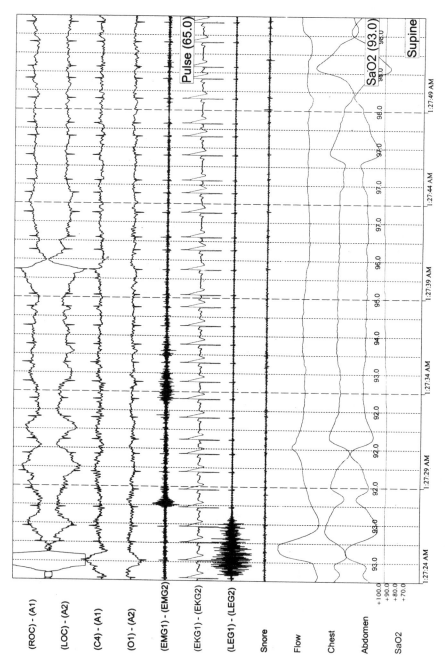

Figure 4. Central sleep apnea. Note the absence of effort in the chest and abdominal channels.

especially true in patients who may have weak respiratory muscles, such as those with neuro-muscular disease. This same patient population is also at risk for central apneas due to the under-lying disease. Therefore, a more sensitive measure of respiratory effort, such as esophageal bal-loon catheter, may be useful to avoid misclassification of apneic episodes.

14. What is the differential diagnosis for central sleep apnea?
    The other main diagnostic consideration is obstructive sleep apnea. Typically, patients with central apnea have less prominent snoring, daytime sleepiness, and obesity. Insomnia may also be more common in central sleep apnea than in obstructive sleep apnea.

15. Describe the diagnostic work-up for patients who present with central sleep apnea.
    The evaluation usually focuses on the cardiac and neurologic systems. An echocardiogram may reveal unsuspected cardiac abnormalities. If a thorough neurologic examination is normal, neuroimaging studies are unlikely to be useful but are still often performed.

PROGNOSIS AND TREATMENT

16. What is the natural history of untreated central sleep apnea?
    The natural history of untreated CSA remains unknown, but it is probably more related to the prognosis of comorbid medical conditions rather than the health consequences of CSA alone.

17. Does the presence of periodic breathing adversely affect the prognosis of patients with comorbid disease?
    The presence of Cheyne-Stokes respiration has been shown to be an independent risk factor for death in patients with congestive heart failure after controlling for other prognostic indicators.

18. What is the mainstay of treatment for central sleep apnea?
    The mainstay of treatment for CSA is treatment or reversal of the underlying disorder. For in-stance, maximal medical therapy for heart failure often improves coexistent CSA and/or CSR-CSA.

19. Discuss the role of CPAP in the setting of CSA or CSR-CSA.
    Some studies have shown a decrease or even resolution of sleep apnea with CPAP therapy, which is somewhat counterintuitive. This finding may occur for several reasons however. Some patients may be misclassified with "central" rather than "obstructive" sleep apnea if respiratory effort is not accurately assessed. It has also been shown that upper airway narrowing and even closure can be found during central apneas, using direct visualization of the airway. CPAP may prevent this phenomenon through increased afferent nerve activity, causing increased tone of the upper airway, or some other similar mechanism.
    It must also be remembered that excessive CPAP levels can actually induce central apneas. Thus, these patients are often difficult to titrate if CPAP is attempted.

20. What is the role of ventilatory assistance in patients with CSA? In which patients may this treatment modality play a role?
    Most sleep specialists reserve this treatment for patients with hypercapnic CSA syndrome. There are multiple modalities for performing this intervention. Originally mechanical ventilation through a tracheostomy was used, but now noninvasive ventilation is most commonly used. This may be done using bilevel positive airway pressure (BiPAP) with or without a "back-up" rate. Negative pressure ventilators, diaphragmatic pacing, and several other methods of ventilatory assistance have also been used.

21. What pharmacologic treatment options are available for central sleep apnea?
    Theophylline, acetazolamide, triazolam, and medroxyprogesterone have been used. The tox-icity of theophylline limits its usefulness; it probably works as a respiratory stimulant. Acetozo-

lamide induces a metabolic acidosis, which then causes a secondary respiratory alkalosis. Only a single study, which used triazoloam, has reported the effects of benzodiazepines. It is thought that the sedative effects decreased the repeated arousal episodes. These patients may be at risk of oversedation, however. Medroxyprogesterone has long been known to act as a respiratory stimulant, but its effects in CSA have not been well studied. It has been studied mainly in obesity-hypoventilation syndrome and appears to be quite efficacious. Unfortunately, it has significant side effects, including gynecomastia, impotence, and decreased libido.

22. What is the role of oxygen in CSA and CSR-CSA?

Supplemental oxygen may alleviate CSA and CSR-CSA caused by altitude or congestive heart failure since reversing the hypoxemia will prevent hyperventilation and thereby stabilize the respiratory system. It is unknown why some patients respond to oxygen whereas others do not. However, most patients at least desaturate less severely with supplemental oxygen.

23. What other gas has been shown to be useful in CSA and CSR-CSA?

Increasing the concentration of inspired carbon dioxide by either increasing the respiratory dead space or rebreathing expired air may decrease central apneas. This effect appears to occur because the carbon dioxide counteracts the hyperventilation, thereby avoiding the secondary hypocapnia and instability in the system.

BIBLIOGRAPHY

1. Bonnet MH, Dexter JR, Arand DL: The effect of triazolam on arousal and respiration in central sleep apnea patients. Sleep 13:31–41, 1990.
2. Bradley TD, Phillipson EA: Central sleep apnea. Clin Chest Med 13:493–504, 1992.
3. Franklin KA, Eriksson P, Sahlin C, Lundgren R: Reversal of central sleep apnea with oxygen. Chest 111(1):163–169, 1997.
4. Hanly PJ, Millar TW, Steljes DG, et al: The effect of oxygen on respiration and sleep in patients with congestive heart failure. Ann Intern Med 111:777–782, 1989.
5. Javaheri S: Central sleep apnea-hypopnea syndrome in heart failure: prevalence, impact and treatment. Sleep 19(10):S229–S231, 1996.
6. Javaheri S: A mechanism of central sleep apnea in patients with heart failure. N Engl J Med 314: 949–954, 1999.
7. Nikkola E, Ekblad U, Ekholm E, et al: Sleep in multiple pregnancy: Breathing patterns, oxygenation, and periodic leg movements. Am J Obstet Gynecol 174:1622–1625, 1996.
8. Sin DD, Logan AG, Fabia SF: Effects of continuous positive airway pressure on cardiovascular outcomes in heart failure patients with and without Cheyne-Stokes respiration. Circulation 102: 61–66, 2000.
9. White DP: Central sleep apnea. In Kryger MH, Roth T, Dement WC (eds): Principles and Practice of Sleep Medicine, 3rd ed. Philadelphia, W.B. Saunders, 2000, pp 827–839.
10. Zolty P, Sanders MH, Pollack IF: Chiari malformation and sleep-disordered breathing: A review of diagnostic and management issues. Sleep 23:637–643, 2000.

10. NARCOLEPSY AND IDIOPATHIC HYPERSOMNOLENCE

Flavia Consens, MD, and Suzanne Stevens, MD

NARCOLEPSY

Epidemiology

1. How common is narcolepsy?
Narcolepsy is not such a rare disease. The prevalence in the United States is roughly 0.05%, although it ranges from 1 in 600 to less than 1 in 10,000. Narcolepsy with cataplexy in the white population occurs in 1 in 4000 people. It is commonly missed, and the delay before diagnosis may be several years.

2. How does the incidence of narcolepsy vary across gender and races?
The overall incidence of narcolepsy is similar for both genders, but it is quite distinct among different ethnic groups. The prevalence is very low in certain populations, as in Israel, where the estimated prevalence is 1 in 500,000. On the contrary, in Japan the prevalence is as high as 1 in 600 people.

3. At what age do most patients present with narcolepsy?
People between 15 and 30 years old are more likely to develop symptoms. The appearance of symptoms before the age of 5 or after the age of 50 is very rare.

4. What is the typical "delay time" before narcolepsy is diagnosed?
Patients typically are symptomatic an average of 15 years before diagnosis.

Pathophysiology

5. What neurochemical disorder causes narcolepsy?
Narcolepsy appears to be caused by the lack of available hypocretins (or orexins), which are neurotransmitters found in the dorsolateral hypothalamus. Either the lack of this neurotransmitter or the deficit of the receptor has been demonstrated in animal models. In humans with narcolepsy, very low levels of hypocretin are found in the cerebrospinal fluid (CSF) of patients with narcolepsy with cataplexy. The hypocretin levels are less consistently abnormal in narcolepsy without cataplexy.

6. What animal models simulate narcolepsy?
There are two: a dog model, with several breeds, and a knockout mice model. Dog models with narcolepsy have mutated receptors for hypocretin 2 that are nonfunctional, whereas in mice abscence of preprohypocretin (a ligand for this receptor) demonstrates sleep abnormalities.

7. How do genes play a role in the animal model of narcolepsy?
In the dog model, narcolepsy is inherited in an autosomal recessive fashion.

8. Is narcolepsy inherited in humans?
The chance that a person with narcolepsy will have an affected offspring is 1–2%, which is 10- to 40-fold higher than the rate in the general population. A familial form of narcolepsy may involve 4–7% of patients.

9. What evidence suggests that narcolepsy may be autoimmune in origin?

Naroclepsy is associated with human leukocyte antigen (HLA) DR2; 90–100% of patients with narcolepsy with cataplexy test positive for HLA DR2. This allele is found on chromosome 6. Many diseases with associated HLA subtypes are autoimmune in origin.

10. What is the most common haplotype in narcoleptic patients?

HLA DQB1*0602 is found in 85–100% of patients having narcolepsy with cataplexy. However, it is found in only 40–60% of patients with narcolepsy without cataplexy. This haplotype has also been found in up to 34% of control subjects, limiting its usefulness.

11. Discuss possible environmental triggers for narcolepsy.

There are reports of head trauma, infections, severe psychological trauma, and disrupted sleep schedules preceding symptoms of narcolepsy.

Diagnosis and Classification

12. What is the tetrad of narcolepsy?

The classical tetrad of narcolepsy consists of excessive daytime sleepiness, cataplexy, hypnagogic or hypnopompic hallucinations, and sleep paralysis. Only 10 to 15% of the patients have this tetrad of symptoms. Most recently, disturbed nocturnal sleep has been added as a "pentad" characteristic of narcolepsy. Clinically, narcoleptics must have at least excessive daytime sleepiness. Automatic behaviors also may be present, but they may be seen in other sleep disorders.

13. Does the excessive daytime sleepiness of narcolepsy differ from sleepiness related to other sleep disorders?

Not necessarily. Excessive daytime sleepiness related to narcolepsy can be preceded by drowsiness or have no precursor, just as with excessive daytime sleepiness related to other sleep disorders such as obstructive sleep apena or insufficient sleep.

14. Define cataplexy.

Cataplexy is a reversible, bilateral muscle weakness of the voluntary muscles, typically triggered by strong emotion such as laughter or anger. Some consider it a necessary component of narcolepsy. Cataplexy may involve limited musculature and be imperceptible to observers or involve the entire musculature, resulting in collapse and potentially serious injury. However, typical cataplectic episodes are manifest as head nodding, jaw sagging, or knee buckling. Cataplexy lasts from seconds to minutes.

15. What happens to deep tendon reflexes during cataplexy?

Deep tendon reflexes are absent during an episode of cataplexy.

16. What happens to level of consciousness during cataplexy?

Consciousness is retained, and patients can recall events during a cataplectic episode, which can help in the differential diagnosis from complex partial seizures or syncope. Some patients may fall asleep immediately after an episode of cataplexy.

17. What emotion is most commonly associated with cataplexy?

Laughter is most commonly associated with cataplexy, although other strong emotions such as anger or fear may trigger episodes as well.

18. What is sleep paralysis?

Sleep paralysis can occur either as the patient is falling asleep or upon awakening. During an episode, people are conscious but unable to move, speak, or open their eyes. This experience can be extremely frightening. Hallucinations may accompany the paralysis. Such episodes can last from seconds to minutes.

19. Define hypnagogic and hypnopompic hallucinations.

They are hallucinatory experiences at sleep onset (hypnagogic) or upon awakening (hypnopompic). They most often involve visual or auditory senses but can also be tactile. Another frequent description is feeling as if the body is floating above the bed (extracorporeal experiences).

20. What do the accessory symptoms of narcolepsy represent neurophysiologically?

Sleep paralysis, hypnagogic hallucinations, and cataplexy are the result of inappropriate intrusion of rapid-eye-movement (REM) sleep.

21. Which symptoms are the most specific and sensitive for narcolepsy?

The most specific symptom is cataplexy, a brief episode of weakness triggered by emotions during which consciousness is preserved. In rare instances, however, cataplexy may be found in other conditions, and there is a rare familial form of cataplexy as well.

22. Are all symptoms present in all narcoleptic patients?

Excessive daytime sleepiness is the only symptom absolutely required for the diagnosis; therefore, it is found in 100% of the patients. Some epidemiologic studies require the presence of cataplexy as a diagnostic feature. Using the current definition, only 60% of patients may have cataplexy, which takes on average 6–7 years to present after the onset of sleepiness.

23. What is the gold standard for the diagnosis of narcolepsy?

Narcolepsy is a clinical diagnosis based on the symptoms and exclusion of other conditions that may account for them.

24. What is the role of the multiple sleep latency test (MSLT) in the diagnosis of narcolepsy?

An MSLT following a nocturnal polysomnogram (to exclude other causes of daytime sleepiness) can provide electrophysiologic evidence supporting the diagnosis of narcolepsy. Typical findings include a mean sleep latency of less than 5 minutes and 2 or more sleep-onset REM periods (SOREMPs) during naps. A MSLT without these features does not exclude the diagnosis of narcolepsy.

25. Can the diagnosis of narcolepsy be made in patients without cataplexy?

Yes. A patient with excessive daytime sleepiness can have the other clinical features (hypnagogic/hypnapompic hallucinations, automatic behaviors, disrupted nocturnal sleep or sleep paralysis) and polysomnographic findings (sleep latency of less than 10 minutes with a REM latency of less than 20 minutes) followed by an MSLT with the criteria described above.

26. Can the diagnosis of narcolepsy be made with genetic testing?

No genetic test is diagnostic for narcolepsy. HLA typing for DQB1*0602 or DR2 has limited value for diagnosis, because is present in 20–35% of the general population. Testing can be useful in atypical cases.

27. Discuss the specificity and sensitivity of the MSLT for diagnosing narcolepsy.

The sensitivity of the MSLT in the diagnosis of narcolepsy is only 60–80%. The finding of SOREMP's in an MSLT is nonspecific, because it can be caused by multiple other conditions, including sleep deprivation, sleep apnea, drug withdrawal, and circadian rhythm disorders, among others.

28. Discuss the role of hypocretin measurement in diagnosing narcolepsy.

At present, measuring CSF levels of hypocretin by lumbar puncture is not routinely done. Hypocretin levels are more consistently low or absent in narcolepsy with cataplexy. Findings in narcolepsy without cataplexy have not been consistent. Blood levels do not correlate with CSF levels in narcolepsy; thus serum tests for hypocretin are not useful.

Prognosis and Treatment

29. Describe the natural history of untreated narcolepsy.

Sleepiness is a lifelong problem, but the other symptoms may fluctuate and tend to improve with age in one-third of patients.

30. Do narcoleptic patients have a normal lifespan?

Yes, with the exception that narcoleptics are more prone to accidents, which may be fatal.

31. What was the earliest treatment for narcolepsy?

Amphetamines were proposed as treatment since the 1930s.

32. What symptom causes the most morbidity in patients with narcolepsy?

Sleepiness causes significant morbidity in all patients. Narcoleptics with severe cataplexy tend to be severely limited by the cataplectic attacks.

33. What medications are approved by the Food and Drug Administration (FDA) for treatment of sleepiness in narcolepsy?

Modafinil was most recently approved for the treatment of sleepiness in narcolepsy. It is a novel stimulant, marketed as a wake-promoting agent, with a different mechanism of action from other stimulants such as amphetamines. It is thought to inhibit dopamine uptake, although it is unknown whether this is the mechanism for improving daytime sleepiness. Additional FDA-approved medications used to treat narcolepsy are methylphenidate and dextroamphetamine. These agents can be used independently or in combination with modafinil to try to minimize the dose of the stimulant medication, which can have many side effects. Pemoline is the only stimulant that is category B in the setting of pregnancy. Other medications used less commonly are protriptyline, monoamine oxidase (MAO) inhibitors, and codeine. Table 1 summarizes these medications.

Table 1. Medications for Treatment of Excessive Daytime Sleepiness in Narcolepsy

MEDICATION	RANGE OF DOSES	FDA-APPROVAL	COMMON SIDE EFFECTS
Modafinil	100–600 mg daily	Yes	Headache
Methylphenidate*	10–60 mg daily	Yes	Tremor, palpitations, irritability, insomnia
Dextroamphetamine*	5–60 mg daily	Yes	Tremor, palpitations, irritability, insomnia
Dexatroamphetamine* and amphetamine	5–60 mg daily	Yes	Tremor, palpitations, irritability, insomnia
Pemoline	37.5–75 mg daily	No	"Black box" warning for liver failure

*Available in extended-release preparation.

34. What medications are used to treat cataplexy?

Antidepressant medications are used to treat cataplexy. Tricyclic antidepressants are effective but have many potential side effects due to their anticholinergic, antihistaminic, and alpha-adrenergic blocking properties. Selective serotonin reuptake inhibitors (SSRIs) can be effective at higher doses. Venlafaxine also has been useful in the treatment of cataplexy. Sodium oxybate (Xyrem) was recently approved by the FDA for the treatment of cataplexy. Table 2 summarizes medications used to treat cataplexy.

Table 2. Medications for Treatment of Cataplexy

MEDICATION	RANGE OF DOSES	FDA-APPROVAL	COMMON SIDE EFFECTS
Sodium oxybate	3–9 mg, taken in 2 doses	Yes	Sedation, nausea
Imipramine	10–100 mg daily	No	Dry mouth, constipation, orthostatic hypotension, drowsiness
Clomipramine	10–150 mg daily	No	Dry mouth, constipation, orthostatic hypotension, drowsiness
Protriptyline	5–60 mg daily	No	Dry mouth, constipation, orthostatic hypotension
Fluoxetine	20–60 mg daily	No	Dry mouth, sexual dysfunction, insomnia
Venlafaxine	37.5–300 mg daily	No	Hypertension, insomnia, nervousness

35. What mechanism is thought to account for the beneficial effect of antidepressant medications in cataplexy?

Decreasing adrenergic uptake appears to be the mechanism responsible for improving cataplexy. Other properties of antidepressants, such as decreasing serotonergic uptake, do not appear to improve cataplexy. This finding possibly accounts for the higher doses of SSRs needed to treat cataplexy, because the higher doses modify the adrenergic system through metabolites. Newer selective adrenergic uptake inhibitors such as reboxetine and atomoxetine may become treatment options in the future.

36. What effects can discontinuing antidepressant medication have on cataplexy?

Abrupt discontinuation of antidepressant medication can cause rebound cataplexy as well as the other REM-related symptoms of narcolepsy, such as sleep paralysis or hypnagogic hallucinations. These medications should be tapered slowly to minimize rebound cataplexy.

37. What medications are approved by the FDA for treatment of cataplexy in narcolepsy?

Most recently sodium oxybate was approved for the treatment of cataplexy. This chemical compound is also called gamma-hydroxybutyrate (GHB), which was known as the "date rape drug" for its intense central nervous system sedative properties. Sodium oxybate is available in a liquid preparation and is dosed once at bedtime with a second dose after approximately 4 hours, which is the approximate duration of action.

38. What behavioral approaches should be considered in treating narcolepsy?

Patients with narcolepsy should be counseled about career choices, and their employers may require education as well. Patients should avoid rotating shiftwork or long stretches of monotonous work without breaks. Jobs requiring driving or operation of heavy equipment should also typically be avoided. The patient may benefit from short naps (15–20 minutes) every 4 hours during the daytime. Additional recommendations are to avoid frequent time zone changes and to maintain regular sleep-wake times in addition to short naps. Although not necessarily behavioral, sensible use of caffeine may also be useful.

39. What other sleep disorders often coexist with narcolepsy?

Periodic limb movement disorder can be seen with narcolepsy or can be induced by antidepressant medication used to treat the cataplexy. However, its contribution to daytime sleepiness is questionable. In addition, REM sleep behavior disorder is seen in up to 10% of narcoleptics.

40. What are future areas of interest in the treatment of narcolepsy?

Hypocretin replacement is a focus of intense research. Animal models using knockout mice and dogs have shown improvement with replacement of hypocretin. This approach holds enormous promise as a future treatment for narcolepsy.

IDIOPATHIC HYPERSOMNOLENCE

Epidemiology

41. How common is idiopathic hypersomnolence?

Idiopathic hypersomnolence (IH) is less common than narcolepsy, with a ratio of 1:10.

42. What is the most common age at presentation? Which gender is most often affected?

Symptoms usually develop during adolescence or young adulthood, without a clear gender preference.

43. When was idiopathic hypersomnolence first described?

IH has been noted since the late 1960s and early 1970s.

Pathophysiology

44. How does the physiology of narcolepsy differ from that of idiopathic hypersomnolence?

The pathophysiology of IH is unknown. It is postulated that a recent viral illness may be a risk factor.

45. Are there any animal models of idiopathic hypersomnolence?

None has been described described at this time.

Diagnosis and Classification

46. What are the diagnostic criteria for idiopathic hypersomnolence?

The diagnosis is made by the initial elimination of other causes of excessive daytime sleepiness. There is usually an insidious onset from weeks to months, typically before age 25, that lasts at least 6 months.

47. How do patients with idiopathic hypersomina present?

Patients often present with long nocturnal sleep episodes and feeling unrefreshed upon awakening. Daytime sleepiness interfering with normal activities is present, and naps are typically long and unrefreshing. This pattern is in contrast to typical naps of narcolepsy, which are usually of short duration (15–20 minutes) and refreshing.

48. Describe the typical polysomnogrpahic findings of idiopathic hypersomnolence.

The polysomnogram (PSG) shows short sleep-onset latency, increased total sleep time, normal sleep architecture, and high sleep efficiency.

49. Is the MSLT useful in the diagnosis of idiopathic hypersomnolence?

Yes. MSLT following a normal PSG that shows a mean sleep latency of less than 10 minutes and less than 2 SOREMPs is supportive of the diagnosis of IH.

Prognosis and Treatment

50. Describe the natural history of untreated idiopathic hypersomnolence,

IH appears to be lifelong, with little variation.

51. Is the prognosis of idiopathic hypersomnolence better or worse than the prognosis of narcolepsy?

Depending on the severity of the sleepiness, IH can be highly disabling. It appears that there are different subgroups of patients with IH, one of which is quite similar to patients with narcolepsy and responds well to stimulants.

BIBLIOGRAPHY

1. Bassetti C, Aldrich MS: Idiopathic hypersomnia: A series of 42 patients. Brain 120 (Pt 8):1423–1435, 1997.
2. Billiard M, Dauvilliers Y: Idiopathic hypersomnia. Sleep Med Rev 5(5):349–358, 2001.
3. Mieda M, Willie JT, Hara J, et al: Orexin peptides prevent cataplexy and improve wakefulness in an orexin neuron-ablated model of narcolepsy in mice. Proc Natl Acad Sci U S A. 2004 March 16 [E publication prior to printed release].
4. Mignot E, Lammers GJ, Ripley B, et al: The role of cerebrospinal fluid hypocretin measurement in the diagnosis of narcolepsy and other hypersomnias. Arch Neurol 59(10):1553–1562, 2002.
5. Overeem S, Mignot E, van Dijk JG, Lammers GJ: Narcolepsy: clinical features, new pathophysiologic insights, and future perspectives. J Clin Neurophysiol 8(2):78–105, 2001.
6. Scammell TE: The neurobiology, diagnosis, and treatment of narcolepsy. Ann Neurol 53:154–166, 2003.
7. Standards of Practice Committee: Practice parameters for the treatment of narcolepsy: An update for 2000. Sleep 24:451–466, 2001.
8. Taheri S, Zeitzer JM, Mignot E: The role of hypocretins (orexins) in sleep regulation and narcolepsy. Annu Rev Neurosci 25:283–313, 2002.
9. Thannickal TC, Moore RY, Nienhuis R, et al: Reduced number of hypocretin neurons in human narcolepsy. Neuron 27:469–474, 2000.

11. CIRCADIAN RHYTHM SLEEP DISORDERS

James K. Wyatt, PhD

1. What modulates sleep propensity, sleep consolidation, and sleep structure?

Sleep initiation, sleep consolidation, and sleep architecture are influenced by the individual effects of and a complex interaction between **sleep homeostatic drive** and the **intrinsic circadian timekeeping system**. For the purposes of the following discussion, the phrase "normal conditions" refers to an adult free of sleep disorders, obtaining a single sleep episode of approximately 8 hours every night, and remaining awake for approximately 16 hours during daylight hours. Intensive, month-long inpatient studies with normal sleepers have demonstrated that under normal conditions, sleep homeostatic pressure allows rapid initiation and consolidation of the first half of the habitual sleep episode. High occurrence of slow-wave sleep and increased power of slow-wave activity during the early part of the sleep episode are thought to reflect the dissipation of sleep homeostatic drive accumulated during the prior wake episode. Consolidation of the second half of the sleep episode results from active promotion of sleep from the circadian system. Circadian drive for sleep peaks at and just after habitual waketime, earning the term **circadian sleep maintenance zone**. Increased duration of REM sleep toward the end of the night results from both active promotion during this circadian phase and **sleep-dependent disinhibition**, the removed competition from slow wave sleep that occurred earlier.

2. What allows a person to maintain alertness at a relatively constant level for 16 hours?

Ease of maintaining wakefulness during the first half of the 16-hour day is achieved primarily through the restorative benefits of the preceding sleep episode and low levels of homeostatic sleep pressure. Mounting homeostatic drive throughout the latter part of the wake episode is counteracted by active promotion of wakefulness from the circadian system. Thus, under normal conditions, it is possible to maintain good alertness and performance for approximately 16 hours due to the consecutive contributions of low homeostatic drive, then circadian wake promotion. Circadian drive for wakefulness peaks a few hours before habitual bedtime, earning the terms **forbidden zone for sleep** or **wake maintenance zone**.

3. Define "optimal" as it pertains to sleep.

In order for optimal sleep and wakefulness to exist as described above, certain conditions must be met. The person must maintain sufficient sustained wakefulness to build up homeostatic pressure. Waketimes and bedtimes must be stable and in agreement with the external light/dark cycle. And the sleep homeostatic and circadian systems must be functioning properly. Violation of any of these conditions is likely to result in one of the six circadian rhythm sleep disorders.

4. What physiologic processes have a circadian rhythm?

Core body temperature reaches its nadir (commonly abbreviated CBTmin) from 1.5 to 2 hours before habitual morning arising time. The pineal hormone melatonin reaches it maximum just before CBTmin. Cortisol has its primary surge in the few hours before habitual waketime.

5. How does light shift circadian phase?

Phototherapy, the prescribed administration of artificial (or naturally occurring) bright light can be used to shift the circadian system to a later (phase-delaying) or earlier (phase-advancing) phase. Phase delays are optimally achieved through phototherapy delivered several hours before CBTmin. Phase advances are optimally achieved through phototherapy timed to occur in the window several hours after the CBTmin.

6. Discuss the key features of delayed sleep phase syndrome.

Typically a disorder of adolescence and early adulthood, delayed sleep phase syndrome (DSPS) is the ability to obtain a sleep episode of satisfactory duration and quality, but only if bedtime (and hence waketime) comes 2 or more hours later than the desired bedtime. The patient complains of sleep-onset insomnia when attempting to initiate sleep during the wake maintenance zone, extreme difficulty in arising early due to the timing of the circadian sleep maintenance zone, and excessive daytime sleepiness due to truncation of the nocturnal sleep episode when not allowed to keep an ad lib schedule.

7. What causes DSPS?

There are various theories about the etiology of DSPS. Clinical lore posits that the circadian system is intact in patients with DSPS but merely "stuck" at a later phase relative to the desired sleep/wake schedule. The sleep-onset complaint is thought to result from attempting to fall asleep during the wake maintenance zone. The difficulty in arising is thought to result from attempting to arise during the circadian sleep maintenance zone. However, behavioral theories can equally well account for DSPS. If a patient remains awake a few hours later than normal under conditions of relatively bright light, a circadian phase delay may occur and be maintained over time. Psychiatric factors may also be at play, including an inability or unwillingness to maintain a regular sleep/wake schedule.

8. Discuss the treatment options for DSPS.

Phototherapy of 1,000–8,000 lux, delivered following the late rising time and gradually moved earlier (e.g., 30 minutes per day), can phase-advance the circadian system. Concurrently, bright light is avoided in the 3-hour window before bedtime to prevent unintentional phase delaying.

Early evening administration of **exogenous melatonin** may phase-advance the circadian system. Alternatively, exogenous melatonin ingested 30 minutes before the desired bedtime may act as a hypnotic, by suppressing the wake-promoting signal from the circadian system encountered maximally during the wake maintenance zone.

As with all circadian rhythm sleep disorders, **rigid adherence to a sleep/wake schedule** is important. Napping must also be avoided or prevented. Daytime naps decrease homeostatic sleep drive and push nighttime sleep onset to a later hour.

9. What is advanced sleep phase syndrome?

The prototypical patient with advanced sleep phase syndrome (ASPS) is an older adult presenting with an inability to remain awake in the evening until the desired bedtime with profound and consistent early morning awakening (EMA) hours before desired wake-up time.

10. Discuss the differential diagnoses for ASPS.

Differential diagnoses for EMA include major depression and rebound following evening alcohol or short-acting hypnotic use. Differential diagnoses for falling asleep too early in the evening include inadequate sleep hygiene, insufficient sleep syndrome, or other conditions expected to produce an increased homeostatic sleep drive (e.g., sleep apnea-hypopnea syndrome).

11. What are the treatment options for ASPS?

Treatment for ASPS involves exposure to bright light in the hours preceding the earlier bedtime, followed by gradually moving the bedtime and the light exposure later (by approximately 30 minutes per day). This approach leads to a gradual delay in circadian phase. Particularly in older patients, an ophthalmologic exam is recommended before bright light exposure is prescribed because of conditions that may lead to lens or retinal damage. Concurrently, the patient must avoid bright light exposure in the 2–3 hours following wake-up time, thereby avoiding a contravening phase advance signal to the circadian system.

12. Discuss the key features of non–24-hour sleep-wake disorder.

The usual complaints of non–24-hr sleep-wake disorder or hypernychthemeral syndrome are (1) a progressively delaying bedtime and waketime if the person is on an ad lib sleep schedule or (2) or waxing and waning episodic insomnia with cycles of weeks to a few months in duration if the person is on a fixed sleep/wake schedule. This disorder can be documented by history and sleep logs/diaries, but actigraphy, which measures movement as a marker of sleep periods, may be a useful diagnostic tool. Figure 1 shows a typical actigraph recording from a patient with non–24-hour sleep-wake disorder.

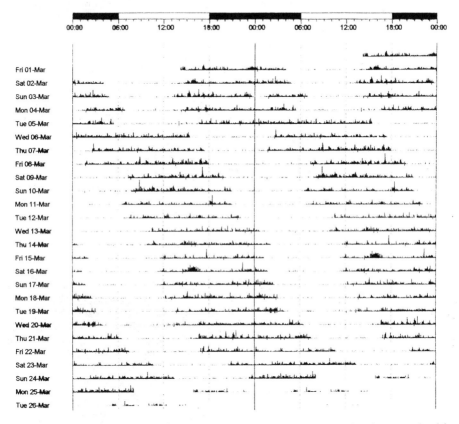

Figure 1. Actigraph recording in a patient with non–24-hour sleep-wake disorder. Note the progressive delay in sleep onset and awake time during the analysis, most evident during the middle of the recording period. Also notice the intermittent attempts to "entrain" or follow a scheduled bedtime and awake time earlier in the recording.

13. What causes non–24-hour sleep-wake disorder?

The simplest explanation for this disorder is functional disconnect between the external light/dark cycle and the circadian system. Without daily phase resetting via photic zeitgebers ("time-givers"), the suprachiasmatic nucleus (SCN) expresses its intrinsic period. As noted above, the intrinsic period has been found to be on average slightly longer than 24 hours in normal subjects; hence, these patients have a progressive delaying of the timing of circadian sleep and wake promotion. The most-studied patient population is the retinally blind, particularly if bilaterally enucleated and thus incapable of transmitting photic input to the SCN. There are also case reports of patients with DSPS who develop a non–24-sleep-wake disorder presentation, highlighting the potential overlap of the two conditions.

14. What are the treatment options for non–24-hour sleep-wake disorder?

In patients with intact visual systems, **strengthening of photic zeitgebers** may allow re-entrainment to the 24-hour day. This approach entails having normal indoor light during the entire waking day and preventing exposure to anything but very dim light (e.g., a night light) during the nighttime sleep episode.

In retinally blind patients, administration of various doses of **exogenous melatonin** has been shown to "phase-lock" or re-entrain free running patients. Details can be found in the references recommended in the bibliography.

As with all circadian rhythm sleep disorders, **rigid adherence to a sleep/wake schedule** is important. Napping must also be avoided or prevented. Daytime naps decrease homeostatic sleep drive and push nighttime sleep onset to a later hour.

A few isolated reports exist of treatment of non-24-hour sleep-wake disorder with **vitamin B$_{12}$**, but it cannot be recommended as a first-line treatment.

15. What is irregular sleep-wake pattern?

Patients with irregular sleep-wake pattern lack the typical monophasic sleep/wake pattern. That is, they do not have a single major nocturnal sleep episode and a major, consolidated daytime wake episode. Behavioral observation or wrist actigraphic monitoring reveals a series of brief (e.g., 2–5 hours) wake episodes followed by brief sleep episodes.

16. What causes irregular sleep-wake pattern?

Investigations in animal models in which the SCN has been lesioned display the disorganized sleep/wake pattern resembling irregular sleep-wake pattern. Humans with this disorder typically have significant pathology of the central nervous system, probably with SCN involvement, perhaps affecting the SCN itself or pathways connecting the SCN to brain regions important for the expression of sleep/wake behavior.

17. Discuss the treatment options for irregular sleep-wake pattern.

In cases of significant, irreversible pathology of the central nervous system, treatment options are limited. Strengthening of the light/dark cycle may allow remaining circadian system constituents to re-establish a wake-promoting signal during daylight hours and a sleep-promoting signal during darkness. To the extent possible, enforcing wakefulness during the daytime allows sufficient build-up of sleep homeostatic pressure to better consolidate and prolong a nighttime sleep episode. Similarly, to the extent possible, enforcing attempts to sleep during the nighttime hours may be beneficial. Mild hypnotics may be helpful, but caution is urged to prevent accidents (e.g., falls) during nighttime awakenings and to lessen the possibility of next-day sedation.

18. What is shift work sleep disorder?

Shift work sleep disorder (SWSD) is a societially driven condition. Modern civilization has determined that value is placed on keeping utility, medical services, police and fire protection, and even goods and service industries operating around the clock. Therefore, in the U.S. work force, millions of workers do not keep to the traditional "nine-to-five" job.

19. Discuss the symptoms of SWSD.

Symptoms of SWSD may include decreased quality and/or quantity of sleep, variable degree of impairment of alertness and performance in the workplace, and a wide range of possible somatic complaints (e.g., gastrointestinal upset, malaise). Economic, safety, health, and quality of life concerns are all pertinent for patients with this SWSD. Shift workers have higher rates of use and abuse of stimulants, ranging from caffeine to prescription and illicit substances as well as alcohol, perhaps used as an hypnotic. Finally, it is commonly reported that the traditional night shift worker obtains 2 hours less daytime sleep than when sleeping at night and not working nights.

20. What are the behavioral treatment options for SWSD?

Working with patients with SWSD to optimize their sleep schedule and minimize cognitive impairment requires a comprehensive knowledge of the patient's sleeping environment, job schedule, and daily activities. Night workers may have to remain awake after returning home in the morning in order to prepare children for school and hence delay sleep onset even further into the circadian wake-promoting zone. Spouses working different shifts may have to arrange common times to meet, placing further restrictions on the timing of sleep. Altering the timing of or responsibility for these home duties can help protect time for sleep.

Ideally, the shift worker should obtain as much sleep as possible in a single, major sleep episode. Those working an early shift (e.g., 4–6 AM start time) should be encouraged to be awake at least 30 minutes before leaving home for work, allowing the potent effects of sleep inertia to clear. Night shift workers should be encouraged to sleep as much as possible immediately after returning home in the morning and to take a prophylactic nap before heading off to work the following night. Controlling environmental factors is also critical in protecting sleep time. Examples include adding light-blocking shades to the bedroom, turning off the telephone, and posting a "day sleeper" or "no solicitors" sign by the doorbell.

21. Discuss other strategies that may help in the treatment of SWSD.

Brief naps (e.g., less than 20 minutes to avoid sleep inertia) at work can provide restorative benefit lasting 2–4 hours. **Modest caffeine intake** may attenuate the expression of sleep homeostatic pressure during the night shift, but it must be consumed early enough in the shift to avoid interfering with subsequent attempts to sleep when returning home in the morning.

Phototherapy has been advocated for shift workers to shift the circadian system to the correct phase relationship with the desired sleep/wake schedule for the shift position. For this approach to function optimally, the worker must remain on the altered sleep/wake schedule on days off (e.g., weekends). However, most shift workers prefer to shift back to a night-sleeping, day-active schedule. Increased illuminance in the workplace may have a beneficial, direct, stimulator effect on arousal independent of the circadian effects.

Exogenous melatonin in the dose range of 1 to 5 mg, taken 30 minutes before going to bed, may allow prolonged daytime sleep in night shift workers. A lower dose, such as 0.1 to 0.3 mg, may aid sleep initiation when the worker attempts to go to bed early to arise for an early morning shift.

22. Define time zone change syndrome.

Time zone change syndrome is roughly synonymous with "jet lag." The circadian- and sleep-related symptoms of jet lag are essentially the same as those encountered in shift work sleep disorder.

23. What cause jet lag?

On arrival at the new location after crossing time zones, the timing of the circadian system is misaligned with the new light-dark cycle and the desired sleep-wake cycle. Many factors can exacerbate this condition. Sleep is commonly restricted before travel because of work demands or home obligations and the need to arise early for morning flights. Furthermore, on long-duration flights, particularly overnight or "red-eye" flights, stress and discomfort make it difficult to obtain the same quality and quantity of sleep that one would attain at home.

24. What are the basic treatment options for jet lag?

Treatments for jet lag can be separated into preflight, inflight, and postflight. The traveler should alleviate any pre-existing sleep debt in the nights before departure and take steps to ensure the minimal level of stress associated with the impending travel (e.g., leaving plenty of time for travel to the airport, packing the night before an early flight). Inflight, the traveler should avoid alcohol and caffeine because of their sleep-disrupting and diuretic effects. Proper hydration can avoid symptoms associated with travel in the relatively low-humidity cabin environment. If the person is unable to obtain an extended major sleep episode on the plane, even brief naps can provide significant restorative value. Finally, upon arrival, the traveler should engage in good sleep hygiene, including trying to maintain their normal bedtime routine, keeping the bedroom quiet and dark, and not engaging in vigorous activity in the hours preceding bedtime.

25. Discuss other treatment approaches to jet lag.

Circadian phase-shifting strategies are beginning to be used in scientific and, unfortunately, casual ways (e.g., internet sales of "jet lag calculators"). Proper timing of exposure to indoor bright light or outdoor sunlight can hasten phase re-entrainment under the new light-dark cycle. However, antidromic or phase shifting in the longer, opposite-of-desired direction can occur in some circumstances. Knowledge of the traveler's preflight sleep/wake cycle allows estimation of the core body temperature minimum (CBTmin), which typically occurs between 90 and 120 minutes before habitual wake-up time. Light exposure in the hours prior to CBTmin shifts phase later, and exposure following CBTmin shifts phase earlier. In the coming years, software may allow the traveler to enter simple sleep diary and itinerary information and obtain a recommendation for times to seek out and avoid light exposure, with the option of preadapting in the days before departure or phase shifting after arrival.

26. Do melantonin and hypnotics have a role in the treatment of jet lag?

As in shift work, oral melatonin may be of use in promoting sleep prior to phase realignment through its suppression of the circadian wake-promoting signal. Low doses should be encouraged, in the range of 0.3 to 5 mg, taken 30 minutes before the desired bedtime. Others may prefer the use of a traditional hypnotic for short-term use while traveling. This is a reasonable alternative to natural sleep or melatonin, as long as the patient has previous experience with and known ability to tolerate the hypnotic with no-to-minimal next-day carryover.

27. How do you collect information to make a diagnosis and monitor treatment for circadian rhythm sleep disorders?

For all of the circadian rhythm sleep disorders, confirmation of the diagnosis and verification of treatment compliance and response are crucial to good care. Maintaining a sleep/wake diary is an inexpensive, reliable way to estimate sleep/wake patterns over a 1- to 2-week interval. For patients who cannot complete this task, use of a wrist actigraph is a great alternative. Through estimation of sleep and wake from monitoring patterns of physical activity, these reusable devices, which cost between $700 and $1500, yield results that agree reasonably with a polysomnogram in terms of total sleep time and slightly less well in terms of sleep latency and number of awakenings. Finally, observer reports may be required to develop convergent validity with the patient's report, particularly for young patients suspected of having DSPS or older patients with ASPS patients or dementia patients with irregular sleep wake pattern.

BIBLIOGRAPHY

1. Ancoli-Israel S, Martin JL, Gehrman P, et al: Effect of light on agitation in institutionalized patients with severe Alzheimer disease. Am J Geriatr Psychiatry 11(2):194-203, 2003.
2. Boulos Z, Campbell SS, Lewy AJ, et al: Light treatment for sleep disorders: Consensus report. VII. Jet lag. J Biol Rhythms 10(2):167-176, 1995.
3. Burgess HJ, Crowley SJ, Gazda CJ, et al: Preflight adjustment to eastward travel: 3 days of advancing sleep with and without morning bright light. J Biol Rhythms 18(4):318-328, 2003.
4. Chesson AL Jr, Littner M, Davila D, et al: Practice parameters for the use of light therapy in the treatment of sleep disorders. Standards of Practice Committee, American Academy of Sleep Medicine. Sleep 22:641-660, 1999.
5. Czeisler CA, Allan J S, Strogatz SH, et al: Bright light resets the human circadian pacemaker independent of the timing of the sleep-wake cycle. Science 233:667-671, 1986.
6. Czeisler CA, Richardson GS, Coleman RM, et al: Chronotherapy: Resetting the circadian clocks of patients with delayed sleep phase insomnia. Sleep 4:1-21, 1981.
7. Czeisler CA, Dumont M, Duffy JF, et al: Association of sleep-wake habits in older people with changes in output of circadian pacemaker. Lancet 340:933-936, 1992.

8. Eastman CI, Boulos Z, Terman M, et al: Light treatment for sleep disorders: Consensus report. VI. Shift work. J Biol Rhythms 10(2):157-164, 1995.
9. Lewy AJ, Bauer VK, Hasler BP, et al: Capturing the circadian rhythms of free-running blind people with 0.5 mg melatonin. Brain Res 918(1-2):96-100, 2001.
10. Monk TH: What can the chronobiologist do to help the shift worker? J Biol Rhythms 15(2):86-94, 2000.
11. Sack RL, Brandes RW, Kendall AR, Lewy AJ: Entrainment of free-running circadian rhythms by melatonin in blind people. N Engl J Med 343(15):1070-1077, 2000.
12. Weitzman ED, Czeisler CA, Coleman RM, et al. Delayed sleep phase syndrome: A chronobiological disorder with sleep-onset insomnia. Arch Gen Psychiatry 38:737-746, 1981.
13. Wyatt JK. Delayed sleepphase syndrome: pathophysiology and treatment options. Sleep, In Press.

12. INSOMNIA

Edward Stepanski, PhD

EPIDEMIOLOGY

1. How is insomnia defined?

Insomnia is present when a patient reports inadequate sleep quantity or sleep quality in conjunction with daytime impairment attributed to deficient sleep. Typically, patients report difficulty with initiating sleep, with maintaining sleep, or with both.

2. How common is insomnia?

Insomnia occurs quite commonly. Survey studies find that about one-third of all adults report difficulty with sleeping at some point in the prior year. About 10% of all adults report that the problem is chronic or severe.

3. When is insomnia considered clinically significant?

The **severity** of daytime impairment determines how aggressively the insomnia should be treated. Some people may report transient reductions in their usual sleep time without any noticeable change in daytime function. In other cases, even apparently small decreases in sleep quantity may be associated with extreme daytime fatigue that impairs the person's ability to maintain work performance, family obligations, or other responsibilities.

The **duration** of the insomnia also determines its clinical significance. An episode of transient insomnia that is present for just a few nights in response to an obvious stressor usually remits spontaneously without intervention. This is not to say that transient insomnia should be ignored. Cases of chronic insomnia start as transient insomnia; therefore, symptomatic treatment may be appropriate to prevent the problem from becoming chronic. In some people, the distress caused by insomnia and behavioral changes in response to insomnia maintain the insomnia until it is a chronic problem. Transient insomnia may also be clinically relevant if it signals another comorbid condition, such as acute psychiatric illness. When insomnia is chronic, occurring on most nights for a period of months, evaluation and treatment are routinely recommended.

4. What are the usual daytime consequences of insomnia?

Fatigue, in conjunction with cognitive and mood changes, is commonly associated with insomnia. Patients report difficulty in concentrating, decreased memory, feelings of irritability, and anhedonia. Some evidence indicates that patients with persistent insomnia are at increased risk to develop major depression. Impairment associated with insomnia can adversely affect occupational and social functioning. Despite reporting fatigue and tiredness, patients with insomnia usually do not have outright sleepiness. That is, patients with insomnia infrequently develop sleepiness of such severity that they fall asleep in the middle of activities. In addition, they often report that if they try to lie down and nap during the day, they are unable to do so. Their difficulty with sleeping appears to be a round-the-clock problem: they are unable to obtain adequate sleep at night and are equally unable to easily obtain recovery sleep during the day.

PATHOPHYSIOLOGY

5. What is known about the neurophysiology of insomnia?

Mechanisms underlying insomnia are not well understood. Various factors that may predispose a person to develop insomnia have been proposed. Patients with insomnia have been shown to have an increased tendency toward physiologic arousal, increased cognitive arousal, and decreased homeostatic sleep drive. Certain patients appear to be more likely to experience insomnia when exposed to a variety of precipitating events (e.g., noisy sleep environment, pain, use of stimulants).

6. Explain the role of stress or traumatic experiences in insomnia.
Increased stress or traumatic experiences can act as precipitating events that trigger an episode of insomnia in a patient who is predisposed to poor sleep.

7. How do I know if a patient is predisposed to insomnia?
Figure 1 depicts a useful theoretical model for understanding chronic insomnia. According to this model, a person has a certain level of predisposition to poor sleep. Insomnia occurs when a precipitating event interacts with this predisposition. Over time, perpetuating factors begin to emerge such that insomnia can continue after the precipitating event remits.

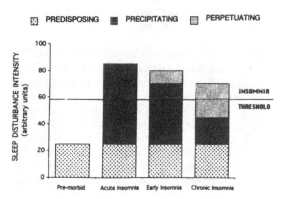

Figure 1. Theoretical model illustrating how predisposing, precipitating, and perpetuating factors can contribute to the development and maintenance of chronic insomnia. (Adapted from Spielman et al: A behavioral perspective on insomnia. Psychiatric Clin North Am 10:541–553, 1987.)

Physiologic hyperarousal and decreased homeostatic drive for sleep are purported to be predisposing factors for the development of chronic insomnia, but this is a controversial area. Any patient with a long history of poor sleep that emerges in response to a variety of precipitating events should be considered to have a high predisposition to poor sleep. Precipitating events in this model are the factors usually targeted in the evaluation of insomnia, such as pain, depression, anxiety, a noisy sleep environment, and jet lag.

Perpetuating factors are typically behavioral and cognitive factors that emerge after a patient has been sleeping poorly for a number of nights. Examples may include changing the sleep-wake schedule to increase time in bed in an effort to accumulate more sleep, increasing use of caffeinated beverages, increasing use of alcohol at bedtime, and worrying during the day about sleep. Appreciating all of these factors, and their relationship to each other is helpful in assuring that all causes of insomnia are targeted for treatment.

DIAGNOSIS AND CLASSIFICATION

8. Describe the classification systems used to categorize insomnia.
Two nosologic systems are used for diagnosing and classifying types of insomnia:
1. The International Classification of Sleep Disorders (ICSD), devised by the American Sleep Disorders Association, is used by sleep specialists. The ICSD has a total of 84 diagnostic categories, with over 12 diagnostic categories that are commonly assigned to a patient presenting with insomnia.
2. The Diagnostic and Statistical Manual-IV (DSM-IV) of the American Psychiatric Association also has a nosologic system for insomnia but contains relatively few categories. The various subtypes described in the ICSD would fit under five broad categories in DSM-IV:

- Primary insomnia
- Insomnia associated with a medical condition
- Insomnia associated with a psychiatric condition
- Insomnia associated with a substance abuse disorder
- Sleep-wake schedule disorder

9. How is insomnia evaluated?

A comprehensive clinical interview is an essential initial step in establishing a diagnosis for a patient presenting with insomnia. This interview is aimed at identifying medical, psychiatric, behavioral, and cognitive factors that may be contributing to poor sleep. In addition, the role of circadian rhythm factors and medication effects must be assessed. Finally, consideration of the possibility of primary sleep disorders, such as periodic limb movement disorder, restless legs syndrome, and sleep-disordered breathing, is needed. An extensive sleep history is critical in the evaluation of patients presenting with insomnia. Typical questions are shown in Table 1. The patient's usual sleep-wake schedule and behavior before bedtime and during the night need to be carefully assessed.

Table 1. *Interview Questions to Obtain a Sleep History for a Patient with Insomnia*

- What do you do prior to bedtime at night?
- When do you get into bed at night?
- Are you watching TV or reading at that time?
- Do you fall asleep with the TV on? If so, when do you turn it off?
- How long does it take you to fall asleep once you turn out the lights?
- Do you sleep through the night, or do you awaken frequently?
- How often do you awaken?
- How long does it take you to return to sleep?
- What do you do when awake at night?
- Do you ever become angry or upset when awake in the middle of the night?
- Do you look at the clock when you awaken during the night?
- Do you ever have something to eat during the night?
- What time do you get out of bed in the morning to start your day?
- How long have you had this sleep pattern?
- How much total sleep do you get per night?
- How much sleep do you need to feel rested during the day?
- How does your sleep-wake schedule change on weekends (or days off)?
- What time did you go to bed and arise before you began to sleep poorly?
- What treatments have you tried for sleep?
- If medication was used, what was the dosage?
- What time did you take it? How long did you take it?
- Did you take it every night? If no, how did you decide which nights you would take it?
- Did you ever take additional medication beyond what was prescribed?
- Did you ever take additional mediation in the middle of the night after awakening?
- How effective was the medication at improving sleep onset? Sleep maintenance?
- Was there any evidence of side effects, such as daytime sedation, motor impairment, or memory impairment?
- Was daytime function improved in any way with use of medication?
- Are you taking medication currently?

10. Why are sleep logs used routinely in the evaluation of insomnia?

Sleep logs provide a more accurate picture of the sleep-wake pattern than a one-time self-report of habitual sleep pattern (see figure in Chapter 7). These data may reveal patterns or variability not apparent from the patient's description of his or her sleep behavior. For example, use of hypnotic medication on an as-needed basis may be sufficiently erratic that it is hard for patients to describe normative behavior in this area.

Sleep logs also help identify other behaviors that may play a role in maintaining insomnia. Once patients begin keeping track of their behavior as required to complete the sleep log, they are often surprised to see the pattern that emerges. For example, they may find that they are drinking eight cups of coffee three or four days per week when they thought that they exceeded four cups on rare occasions. Or they may find that their worst nights of sleep occur on nights when they argue with a spouse or visit their sick parents. All of this information is helpful in understanding the triggers for insomnia in a specific patient.

11. When is polysomnography indicated for the evaluation of insomnia?

In cases of insomnia, a diagnosis can usually be made on the basis of a clinical interview. Therefore, polysomnography is generally recommended only when a primary sleep disorder (e.g., periodic limb movement disorder [PLMD], obstructive sleep apnea [OSA]) is suspected. Definitive diagnosis of PLMD or OSA requires polysomnographic documentation. Polysomnography should also be considered when the insomnia is refractory to standard treatment approaches and significant daytime impairment is reported. Another insomnia diagnosis aided by polysomnographic data is sleep-state misperception. In this condition, the patient reports obtaining little or no sleep despite obtaining normal sleep times on objective testing.

12. How is actigraphy used in the evaluation of insomnia?

Actigraphy measures physical activity with a portable device (usually including an accelerometer) worn on the wrist. Actigraphy provides an estimate of total sleep time and sleep efficiency that can be useful in evaluating the severity of insomnia or the patient's progress in response to treatment. Actigraphy may also be used to assess a patient's adherence to treatment recommendations (e.g., keeping a specific sleep-wake schedule). Advantages of actigraphy are its low cost, especially compared with other objective measures of sleep such as polysomnography, and its ability to collect data continuously over consecutive nights and weeks. Night-to-night variability is common in patients with insomnia; therefore, a large sample of nights provides a more precise understanding of the sleep pattern than can be obtained by studying a single night.

PROGNOSIS AND TREATMENT

13. Describe the typical outcome of acute insomnia.

Almost everyone experiences an episode of insomnia at some point, and most people have several episodes over the course of their lifetime. Generally these episodes remit spontaneously. However, in people predisposed to poor sleep, episodes of acute insomnia may recur frequently and take longer to resolve or require intervention. Eventually, these patients may develop chronic insomnia.

14. Describe the typical outcome of chronic insomnia.

Treatment outcome studies show that about two-thirds of patients with insomnia can obtain normal sleep with treatment (see discussion of treatment approaches below). Patients who develop chronic insomnia are believed to have a predisposition to poor sleep and therefore are always somewhat more likely to experience poor sleep when exposed to precipitating factors. Such patients can learn behavioral techniques to improve sleep; they also can learn to avoid exposure to factors that act as triggers of insomnia. However, even with successful treatment, such people are still at increased risk for occasional episodes of insomnia.

15. What are the main forms of treatment for patients with insomnia?

There are two types of treatment for primary insomnia: cognitive-behavioral therapy and pharmacologic treatment. Both are described in detail below. Other treatment approaches may be used when insomnia is deemed to be secondary to another primary disorder. For example, if insomnia appears to be secondary to a major depressive disorder, treatment for depression is needed to treat the insomnia. When insomnia is associated with pain in a patient with osteoarthritis, treatment may consist of more aggressive therapy for pain during the night.

16. Define cognitive-behavioral therapy.

Cognitive-behavioral therapy (CBT) is an umbrella term that refers to a number of different treatments that employ changes in behavior or cognition to improve sleep. Behavioral treatments used for insomnia include sleep restriction therapy, stimulus control therapy, and progressive muscle relaxation. Each of these approaches requires that the patient receive instruction in how to change behavior and adhere to new sleep habits. Cognitive therapy seeks to eliminate irrational beliefs about sleep and fears of not sleeping.

17. On what theories are cognitive-behavioral treatments based?

- Stimulus control therapy
- Sleep restriction therapy
- Progressive muscle relaxation
- Cognitive therapy

18. Explain stimulus control therapy.

Stimulus control therapy (SCT) is based on principles of classic conditioning from learning theory. The underlying assumption of conditioned insomnia is that by pairing waking activities with the sleep environment, the sleep environment becomes a discriminative cue for increased arousal and wakefulness. When a patient with insomnia enters the bedroom, he or she sees the bedroom clock and other cues that lead to increased tension. The goal of SCT is to pair a feeling of drowsiness and sleep with the sleep environment and to break the negative conditioning. This goal is accomplished by having the patient spend time in bed only when he or she is drowsy or asleep.

19. How does sleep restriction therapy work?

Sleep restriction therapy seeks to improve sleep consolidation by limiting the time available for sleep and increasing the homeostatic drive for sleep. Patients become more sleepy during the day as this treatment progresses, and this pattern translates to shorter sleep latencies at night and increased sleep efficiency. Eventually time in bed is increased as long as the sleep remains consolidated.

20. Explain the goals of progressive muscle relaxation.

Progressive muscle relaxation is one of many therapies that are aimed at reducing somatic and cognitive arousal in order to promote a shorter latency to sleep. Relaxation treatments are based on the premise that patients with insomnia have elevated levels of tension and arousal that are incompatible with sleep. Other examples of relaxation-based treatments include meditation, guided imagery, and self-hypnosis.

21. How is cognitive therapy used to treat insomnia?

Cognitive therapy is based on the observation that worry about sleep leads to increased anxiety and excessive cognitive arousal that interfere with the ability to sleep. This approach teaches patients to identify when they are exaggerating the significance of their difficulty with sleep and helps them to develop other responses that do not lead to anxiety and panic. For example, when awake during the night, patients with insomnia commonly worry that they will be unable to perform job responsibilities during the following day. As a result, they fear that they may lose their job or suffer some other extreme misfortune as a consequence of being unable to return to sleep immediately. In reality, they are likely to have had numerous occasions when they went to work after having had much less sleep than they would have preferred. On those past occasions, they compensated for the night of short sleep and performed their responsibilities as needed. It is important not to trivialize the significance of the patient's suffering during the day following nights of insomnia. The goal of this therapy is to place the consequences of insomnia into a rational context so that concerns about sleep are in proportion to the problem.

22. Has the effectiveness of cognitive behavioral therapy been proved in clinical trials?

The efficacy of various CBT approaches in the treatment of insomnia has been demonstrated in clinical trials by Morin et al. in 1999 and Edinger et al. in 2001. CBT has been compared with pharmacologic treatment and placebo treatments. CBT shows short-term improvement equivalent to pharmacologic treatment, but it is superior to pharmacologic treatment at long-term follow-up.

23. What is meant by the term *sleep hygiene*?

Sleep hygiene refers to a set of factors that are required for maintenance of a normal sleep-wake pattern. Sleep hygiene recommendations have varied over the years, but common examples include maintenance of a regular sleep-wake schedule, limiting use of caffeine and alcohol, avoiding naps, eliminating noise and light from the sleep environment, and not looking at the clock during the night.

24. Why is sleep hygiene thought to be important in the pathophysiology of insomnia?

Following appropriate sleep hygiene rules is seen as necessary, but not sufficient, for establishing a normal sleep-wake pattern. Therefore, establishing good sleep hygiene is generally part of the treatment plan for any patient presenting with insomnia. It is also relevant because violations of sleep hygiene become more common once a person has started to encounter sleep problems. When sleep is poor, people often compensate in ways that further increase the likelihood of continued insomnia. For example, after a night of poor sleep, people may stay in bed later to try and get additional rest, lie down to nap during the day, or drink extra cups of coffee. These changes may help them feel better at the moment but decrease the likelihood of restoring a normal sleep-wake schedule on subsequent nights.

25. What classes of drugs have been used to treat insomnia?

Many classes of drugs with sedating properties are commonly used to treat insomnia. "Sleeping pills" include benzodiazepine compounds as well as newer nonbenzodiazepines such as imazopyridines. Sedating antidepressants are often used in the treatment of insomnia. These medications are believed to be safer by some practitioners because they are unlikely to be abused. However, since use of anti-depressants as a treatment for insomnia is an off-label use, the dose-response relationship has often not been established for treatment of insomnia.

26. What are the pharmacologic properties of the most common compounds used for treatment of insomnia?

Compounds commonly used to treat insomnia differ with respect to duration of action, rate of absorption, and side-effect profile (Table 2). There has been a trend toward use of shorter-acting hypnotic medications to avoid residual daytime sedation.

Table 2. *Characteristics of Medications Used for Sleep*

Generic Name	Trade Name	Duration of Action	Half-Life (hrs)	Maximum Dose Recommended
Clonazepam	Klonopin	Long	> 24	2 mg
Estazolam	ProSom	Intermediate	17.1	2 mg
Eszopiclone	Estorra	Short	5	
Flurazepam	Dalmane	Long	40–103*	30 mg
Quazepam	Doral	Long	> 24	15 mg
Temazepam	Restoril	Intermediate	8.4	30 mg
Triazolam	Halcion	Short	2.6	0.25 mg
Zaleplon	Sonata	Short	1.0	10 mg
Zolpidem	Ambien	Short	1.5	10 mg

* For active metabolites.

27. Are short-acting or long-acting sedative/hypnotic agents preferred?

Selection of a short- or long-acting hypnotic medication should be based on the clinical characteristics of the individual patient. In general, patients initially require a medication that allows them to fall asleep faster and also to return to sleep if they awaken during the night. However, residual sedation during the following day is usually unwanted. Therefore, short- or intermediate-acting medications are almost always preferable to long-acting medications. One exception is the patient who has an anxiety disorder for which daytime sedation is therapeutic. Use of a long-acting compound at bedtime (e.g., clonazepam) may help with insomnia as well as daytime anxiety so that additional anxiolytic medication during the day is unnecessary.

28. What are the most common side effects of sedative/hypnotic compounds?

Impairments in psychomotor performance and memory occur with sedation. These effects are limited to the period of sedation; therefore, long-acting compounds may produce these effects into the following day. This pattern is called residual sedation, and when it occurs, patients complain of having a morning "hangover." A "hangover" or grogginess in the morning is one effect that may lead patients to abandon treatment. Residual sedation should be assessed after beginning pharmacologic treatment because it may compromise patient safety.

29. Define rebound insomnia.

Rebound insomnia occurs when a patient discontinues a hypnotic medication and experiences insomnia that is worse than at baseline. It is expected that insomnia may return to the baseline level of severity once the hypnotic medication is removed; thus, rebound insomnia is present only when sleep is worse than at baseline. The tendency to experience rebound insomnia is heightened with use of short-acting compounds. Duration of use also increases the likelihood of rebound, but rebound can occur after only one night of administration. Individual differences play a role in this phenomenon. Some patients experience severe rebound routinely with drug discontinuation, whereas others appear to have only occasional mild difficulty with discontinuation. Rebound insomnia has not been shown to last more than a couple nights. Tapering the dose for a few nights prior to discontinuation has been shown to eliminate the risk of rebound insomnia.

BIBLIOGRAPHY

1. American Psychiatric Association: Diagnostic and Statistical Manual of Mental Disorders, 4th ed. Washington, DC, American Psychiatric Association, 1994.
2. American Sleep Disorders Association: The International Classification of Sleep Disorders, Revised: Diagnostic and Coding Manual. Rochester, MN, American Sleep Disorders Association, 1997.
3. Edinger JD, Wohlgemuth WK, Radtke RA, et al: Cognitive behavioral therapy for treatment of chronic primary insomnia: A randomized controlled trial. JAMA 285:1856–1864, 2001.
4. Mendelson WB: Hypnotics: Basic mechanisms and pharmacology. In Kryger M, Roth T, Dement W (eds): Principles and Practice of Sleep Medicine, 3rd ed. Philadelphia, W.B. Saunders, 2000, pp 407–413.
5. Morin CM: Insomnia: Psychological Assessment and Management. New York, Guilford Press, 1993.
6. Morin C, Colecchi C, Stone J, et al: Behavioral and pharmacological therapies for late-life insomnia. JAMA 281:991–999, 1999.
7. Stepanski E: Etiology of insomnia. In Lee-Chiong T, Sateia M, Carskadon M (eds): Sleep Medicine. Philadelphia, Hanley & Belfus, 2002, pp. 161–168.
8. Stepanski EJ, Wyat JK: Use of sleep hygiene in the treatment of insomnia. Sleep Med Rev 7: 215–225, 2003.

13. RAPID-EYE-MOVEMENT PARASOMNIAS

Suzanne Stevens, MD

RAPID-EYE-MOVEMENT BEHAVIOR DISORDER

Epidemiology

1. What is the prevalence of rapid-eye-movement behavior disorder in the general population?

In the general population, the prevalence of rapid-eye-movement behavior disorder (RBD) is 0.5%. However, there is a higher prevalence in patients with neurodegenerative processes.

2. What neurodegenerative diseases are associated with RBD?

Parkinson's disease, Lewy body disease, and Parkinson plus syndrome have a high prevalence of RBD.

3. Which gender has a higher prevalence of RBD?

In large series, up to 87% of patients have been males.

4. Does RBD ever precede the onset of Parkinson disease?

Of patients diagnosed with idiopathic RBD, approximately one-third have been reported to eventually develop Parkinson's disease. Some reports have suggested that this number is higher.

5. What is the typical age of a patient with RBD?

The mean age has varies from 52 to 61 years (range: 9–84 years) in large series of patients with RBD.

Pathophysiology

6. Is there an animal model for RBD?

In 1965, Jouvet developed a feline model of RBD, in which lesions of the perilocus coruleus region of the pons resulted in motor activity during REM sleep. Spontaneously occurring RBD activity has been reported in cats and dogs.

Diagnosis and Classification

7. How do patients with RBD typically present?

Sleep-related injury has been the presenting complaint in up to 79% of patients. Injuries attributed to RBD include ecchymoses, lacerations, and fractures, including subdural hematoma. The bed partner is at risk for injury as well.

8. What happens to the dream content of patients with RBD?

Dreams are described as more vivid and intense and often have the theme of being attacked or protecting against an aggressor. When acting out these dreams, the patient is dreaming that he is attacking an aggressor, but in actuality he may be attacking the bed partner.

9. What typically happens if the patient with RBD is awakened during an episode of RBD?

Typically the patient is immediately oriented and often can recall dream content that matches the motor activity demonstrated.

10. What are the diagnostic criteria for RBD?

The International Classification of Sleep Disorders (ICSD) lists the criteria for RBD as follows. The minimal criteria required for diagnosis are B plus C:

A. The patient has a complaint of violent or injurious behavior during sleep.
B. Limb or body movement is associated with dream mentation.
C. At least one of the following occurs:
    a. Harmful or potentially harmful sleep behaviors
    b. Dream appears to be "acted out"
    c. Sleep behaviors disrupt sleep continuity
D. Polysomnographic monitoring demonstrates at least one of the following:
    a. Excessive augmentation of chin electromyographic (EMG) tone
    b. Excessive chin or limb phasic EMG activity and one or more of the following:
        i. Excessive limb or body jerking
        ii. Complex, vigorous, or violent behaviors
        iii. Absence of epileptic activity in association with the disorder
E. The symptoms are not associated with mental disorders but may be associated with neurologic disorders.
F. Other sleep disorders (e.g., sleep terrors or sleep walking) can be present but are not the cause of the behavior.

11. Is a sleep study required for diagnosis of RBD?

Polysomnography (PSG) is not required according to the minimum criteria of the ICSD. However, some sleep specialists believe that polysomnography is mandatory given the potential for injury. Figure 1 shows a typical polysomnogram recording during an episode of RBD.

12. What are possible causes for the acute development of RBD?

Acute RBD may be associated with withdrawal from alcohol, withdrawal from REM-suppressing medications, or drug addiction.

13. What diseases are associated with the chronic form of RBD?

Chronic RBD is either idiopathic or associated with neurologic disease.

14. What typically occurs to the sleep architecture (particularly REM sleep) in patients with RBD?

REM latency, percent REM of total sleep time, and number and periodicity of REM periods remain intact.

15. What is the prevalence of psychiatric disorders among patients with RBD?

In large series of patients described with RBD, the prevalence of lifetime psychiatric disease was 25–35%, which is thought to be similar to that of the general population.

16. What is the differential diagnosis of RBD?

The differential diagnosis of RBD includes nocturnal seizures, rhythmic movement disorder, and disorders of arousal (e.g., confusional arousal, sleepwalking, sleep terrors). Movements associated with obstructive apneas can cause motor activity similar to that seen in RBD, as can any disorder causing arousals during sleep such as periodic limb movement disorder. Other diagnoses in the differential include nocturnal panic disorder, dissociative disorders, and malingering.

17. What is the parasomnia overlap syndrome?

The parasomnia overlap syndrome can present as a history consistent with sleepwalking or sleep terrors but with motor disinhibition during both NREM and REM sleep.

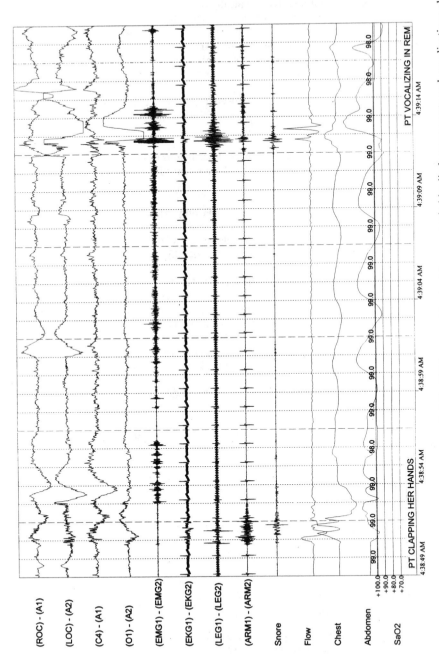

Figure 1. A typical epoch of RBD showing lack of REM atonia (chin EMG, arm and leg leads) accompanied by limb movements and vocalizations observed by the technician.

Prognosis and Treatment

18. During what time of night does RBD typically occur?
RBD typically occurs in the last half of the night when the majority of REM sleep occurs.

19. What are the polysomnographic findings of RBD?
REM sleep without atonia, accompanied by motor activity or vocalizations, is polysomnographic evidence of RBD.

20. What happens to the heart rate during the enactment of a dream in RBD?
Tachycardia may not be present during motor movements, possibly reflecting the decreased sympathetic activity expected during REM sleep.

21. What types of neurologic lesions have been described as causing secondary RBD?
Plaques associated with multiple sclerosis and brainstem stroke have resulted in secondary RBD.

22. How should patients with RBD modify their sleeping environment?
Securing the sleep environment to minimize the risk of injury is mandatory in advising patients with RBD. Objects that pose a danger should be removed from the room. Mattresses may be placed on the floor and surrounded with pillows, if needed.

23. What pharmacologic treatments may be used for RBD?
Clonazepam has been shown to be 90% effective in a population able to take it over the long term. Clonazepam has been reported to improve both motor sleep behaviors and nightmares within 1 week of beginning therapy at a dose of 0.5 mg at bedtime, increasing to 1.0 mg if needed. Other medications reported in the literature and anecdotally but not studied systematically include carbmazepine, carbodipa/levodopa, gabapentin, monoamine oxidase inhibitors, desipramine, melatonin, clonidine, triazolam, and clozapine. Other benzodiazepines may also be effective.

24. What have been the polysomnographic findings in patients with RBD treated with clonazepam?
The sleep architecture remains the same, and atonia is observed during REM sleep, but without gross motor movements, indicating that perhaps clonazepam works on the motor system independently from the REM atonia system. This effect is possibly due to the serotinergic activity of clonazepam.

25. What are the typical findings on MRI of idiopathic RBD?
Subcortical small vessel disease has been seen in some patients with idiopathic RBD.

REM-ASSOCIATED SUSTAINED NOCTURNAL PENILE ERECTIONS

26. Who at risk for sustained nocturnal penile erections?
Middle-aged or older men.

27. How common is this disorder?
The prevalence is unknown.

27. What is thought to be the mechanism of this disorder?
The mechanism is unknown. Evaluation of the penis is typically normal.

28. How do patients with sustained nocturnal penile erections present?
Patients present with the complaint of penile pain during erections that usually occur during REM sleep, resulting in awakenings. Daytime erections are reported to be normal.

29. Are REM-associated sustained penile erections a persistent or self-limited disease?
Although in general the course for this disorder is unknown, the condition can worsen with time.

30. Are there any proven treatments for sleep-related painful erections?
There are anecdotal reports of treatment with clozapine, propranolol, and paroxetine.

REM SLEEP-RELATED SINUS ARREST

31. In what population is REM sleep-related sinus arrest seen?
Young adults of either gender who are otherwise healthy.

32. How common is REM sleep-associated sinus arrest?
Because of the few cases described, prevalence is not known.

33. What are the findings on the PSG?
Clusters of sinus arrest during REM sleep are seen, lasting up to 9 seconds. These clusters can recur repeatedly throughout REM.

34. What are findings on cardiac evaluation?
Prolonged electrocardiographic monitoring demonstrates sinus arrest exclusively during REM sleep. Electrocardiographic and angiographic findings during wakefulness are unrevealing.

35. What are the ICSD criteria for the diagnosis of REM sleep-related sinus arrest?
Minimal criteria are the following:
1. The patient has no related sleep complaint.
2. PSG monitoring demonstrates asystole, lasting greater than 2.5 seconds and occurring solely during REM sleep.
3. There is no evidence of medical disorders accounting for the cardiac arrhythmia.
4. There is no evidence for other sleep disorders (e.g., sleep apnea/hypopnea syndrome) to account for the cardiac arrhythmia.

BIBLIOGRAPHY

1. Boeve BF, Silber MH, Ferman TJ: Association of REM sleep behavior disorder and neurodegenerative disease may reflect an underlying synucleinopathy. Move Disord 16:622–630, 2001.
2. Comella CL, Nardine TM, Diederich NJ, Stebbins GT: Sleep-related violence, injury and REM sleep behavior disorder in Parkinson's disease. Neurology 51:526–529, 1998.
3. Culebras A, Moore JT: Magnetic resonance findings in REM sleep behavior disorder. Neurology 39:1519–1523, 1989.
4. Ferini-Strambi L, Oldani A, Zucconi M, et al: Cardiac autonomic activity during wakefulness and sleep in REM sleep behavior disorder. Sleep 19:367–369, 1996.
5. Lapierre O, Montplaisir J: Polysomnographic features of REM sleep behavior disorder: Development of a scoring method. Neurology 42:1371–1374, 1992.
6. Olson EJ, Boeve BF, Silber MH: Rapid eye movement sleep behaviour disorder: demographic, clinical and laboratory findings in 93 cases. Brain 123:331–339, 2000.
7. Schenck CH, Mahowald MW: REM sleep behavior disorder: Clinical, developmental, and neuroscience perspectives 16 years after its formal identification. Sleep 25:120–138, 2002.

14. NON-RAPID-EYE-MOVEMENT PARASOMNIAS

Suzanne Stevens, MD, and Damien Stevens, MD

SLEEPWALKING

1. What is another name for sleepwalking?
Somnambulism, which comes from the Latin words *somnus* (sleep) and *ambulare* (to walk), is the medical term for sleepwalking.

2. What is the most common age for sleepwalking?
It is most common in children aged 4 to 6 years but can persist into adulthood. Adult-onset sleepwalking is rare.

3. In what stage of sleep does sleepwalking typically occur?
Most sleepwalking episodes occur in slow-wave sleep, stage 3 or 4. Occasionally sleepwalking occurs during stage 2 sleep.

4. At what time of night does sleepwalking typically occur?
Episodes usually occur during the first or second cycle of slow-wave sleep, which is typically in the first third of the night.

5. What are precipitating factors for sleepwalking?
Precipitating factors include sleep deprivation, stress, and pain. Other primary sleep disorders that interrupt sleep, such as sleep apnea, may trigger sleepwalking as well.

6. What treatment options are available for sleepwalking?
The vast majority of children outgrow sleepwalking. However, in patients who harm themselves or have persistent episodes the first step is to avoid triggers or precipitating factors such as sleep deprivation. Making the sleep environment safe is also essential to decrease the chance for injury. Safety strategies may include locks on doors, alarms, and safeguarding of sharp objects. Some patients may benefit from pharmacologic therapy

7. What are the pharmacologic treatments for sleepwalking?
The most common therapy is benzodiazepines, which are known to suppress slow-wave sleep, but tricyclic antidepressants are also used. Medications are usually used only for short periods during frequent episodes.

SLEEPTALKING

8. What is the medical term for sleeptalking?
Somniloquy, which comes from the Latin words *somnus* (sleep) and *loqui* (to speak).

9. What stage of sleep is most commonly associated with sleeptalking?
Most commonly sleeptalking occurs in stages 1 and 2 and REM sleep. Rarely sleeptalking occurs in slow-wave sleep.

10. What is the natural history of sleeptalking?
The course is typically benign; treatment is rarely required.

CONFUSIONAL AROUSALS

11. What is another term for confusional arousals?

Sleep drunkenness was the original term for confusional arousals.

12. How common are confusional arousals?

Few data about the actual incidence or prevalence are available, but confusional arousals are common in young children, especially before the age of 5 years. The prevalence decreases with age. Confusional arousals are uncommon in adults, but once again the actual incidence is unknown.

13. What causes confusional arousals?

The cause remains unknown; in rare cases, a central nervous system lesion is found.

14. Which patients most commonly have confusional arousals?

The rate in males and females is similar, but there is a strong familial pattern with an increased presence in certain families. No genetic markers have been described. Confusional arousals often coexist in patients with sleepwalking and sleep terrors.

15. What is required for the diagnosis of confusional arousals?

Confusion during and after an arousal from sleep is the only essential element of the diagnosis. This confusion may consist of disorientation, slow speech, decreased mentation, inappropriate behavior, and decreased responsiveness. Episodes usually occur earlier in the night and during slow-wave sleep. Polysomnography (PSG) is not required for the diagnosis.

16. Do patients with confusional arousals recall the episode?

Patients typically have no recall of the episode or only minimal fragments of recall.

SLEEP TERRORS

17. What is the medical term for sleep terrors?

The Latin term is *pavor nocturnus*, which translates into night terror.

18. How common are sleep terrors?

Sleep terrors are more common in children than adults with a prevalence of approximately 3% and 1%, respectively.

19. Which patients most commonly develop sleep terrors?

Sleep terrors are more common in children than adults and in males than females. Coexistent psychopathology may be seen in adults but typically not in children.

20. In which stage of sleep do sleep terrors usually occur?

They usually occur in slow-wave sleep and in the first third of the night.

21. How is a typical sleep terror episode described?

Episodes usually begin with an intense scream or cry. Patients demonstrate increased autonomic activity with typical findings of tachycardia, tachypnea, diaphoresis, hypertension, and increased muscle tone.

22. How are night terrors different from nightmares?

Patients with nightmares typically recall dreaming, whereas episodes of sleep terror are associated with total or at least partial amnesia. If a complete arousal occurs, patients with sleep terrors are often confused, whereas nightmares do not cause confusion.

RHYTHMIC MOVEMENT DISORDER

23. What are other names for rhythmic movement disorder?
The Latin term *jactatio capitis nocturna* (nocturnal banging of the head) is considered a synonym, although it specifically refers to the head-banging form of rhythmic movement disorder.

24. Which patient group most commonly develops rhythmic movement disorder?
Rhythmic movement disorder is most common in infants and young children. There is a genetic component with increased prevalence in twins and families. It is also more common in males than females with a ratio of 4:1.

25. What "movements" are typically seen in rhythmic movement disorder?
Typical movements seem to vary with age. Body-rocking has a mean onset of 6 months, head-banging a typical onset of 9 months, and head-rolling 10 months. Head-banging is the most common form of movement.

26. How fast are the movements in most patients?
The frequency varies significantly, but the rate is usually between 0.5 to 2 cycles per second.

27. How common is rhythmic movement disorder?
It is estimated that up to two-thirds of 9-month-old children have some form of rhythmic movement disorder. New onset rhythmic movement disorder in adults is rare.

28. Describe the natural history of rhythmic movement disorders.
By the age of 18 months the rate falls to half the prevalence at 9 months. Most patients outgrow the movements by age 4, years with a prevalence of only 8%. If the disorder persists past the age of 10 years, mental retardation, autism, or another developmental disorder may be present.

29. In which stage of sleep do the movements typically occur?
Few PSG studies exist, but most movements occur in light non-REM sleep, stage 1 or 2 sleep. However, movements have been recorded in slow-wave sleep and rarely even in REM sleep.

30. What are the potential complications of rhythmic movement disorder?
Scalp lacerations, bruises, subdural hematoma, retinal petechiae, and skull callus formation have been reported. Carotid dissection has also been described due to head-banging.

31. What treatment options are available for rhythmic movement disorder?
Most patients outgrow the movements without any specific treatment. Occasionally, sleep is disrupted severely enough to warrant treatment. This scenario is rarely true in children but possible in adults. The few case reports note a fairly good response to benzodiazepines or antidepressants.

NOCTURNAL EATING

32. What is nocturnal or night eating?
Nocturnal eating consists of recurrent arousals during the sleep period and inability to return to sleep without eating or drinking. Typically large amounts of food are consumed. Note that the patient awakens; the eating does not occur during a sleepwalking or confusional arousal episode. The patient may report awareness of the episode, but amnesia is occasionally reported. In the childhood form of this disorder, caretakers may play a role in the pathogenesis. An adult form is also recognized, but the pathogenesis may be different.

33. How common is nocturnal eating?
Very few patients have been reported in the medical literature, but the prevalence is unknown. Some believe that a significant number of patients seen in obesity clinics have this disorder.

34. Is sleep "normal" in patients with nocturnal eating?

Once again, few data are available to answer this question. Preliminary evidence suggests that the sleep/wake cycle is normal except for increased arousals. Some researchers believe that a circadian disorder may also play a role, causing hunger at an abnormal time. This theory, however, remains unproved.

35. What are indications for PSG in the setting of nocturnal eating?

No clear consensus exists, but most clinicians agree that violent or injurious behavior, excessive daytime somnolence, or stereotypic behavior raises the possibility of a seizure disorder and suggests the need for PSG. Extended electroencephalographic (EEG) monitoring may also be warranted if seizures are suspected.

36. What behavioral treatment options are available for night eating?

The main goal is to make food inaccessible, thereby decreasing the possibility of night eating or at least decreasing the caloric intake. No clinical trials of the success rate for this intervention have been reported, but it is an obvious, simple, and inexpensive first step.

37. What pharmacologic treatments are available for night eating?

Preliminary results from an open-label study suggest that sertraline may reduce nocturnal eating episodes. Other anecdotal treatments include fluoxetine and buproprion. Clonazepam has been used as well. No blinded, randomized trials have been reported for this disorder.

BIBLIOGRAPHY

1. Hublin C, Kaprio J, Partinen M, et al: Parasomnias: Co-occurrence and genetics. Psychiatr Genet. 11(2):65–70, 2001.
2. Mahowald MW, Schenck CH: NREM sleep parasomnias. Neurol Clin 14:675–696, 1996.
3. Malow BA: Paroxysmal events in sleep. J Clin Neurophysiol 19:522–34, 2002.
4. Ohayon MM, Guilleminault C, Priest RG: Night terrors, sleepwalking, and confusional arousals in the general population: Their frequency and relationship to other sleep and mental disorders. J Clin Psychiatry 60:268–276, 1999.
5. Schenck CH, Mahowald MW: Review of nocturnal sleep-related eating disorders. Int J Eat Disord 15:343–356, 1994.
6. Schenck CH, Mahowald MW: Parasomnias. Managing bizarre sleep-related behavior disorders. Postgrad Med 107(3):145–156, 2000.
7. Spaggiari MC, Granella F, Parrino L, et al: Nocturnal eating syndrome in adults. Sleep 17: 339–344, 1994.
8. Zucconi M, Ferini-Strambi L: NREM parasomnias: Arousal disorders and differentiation from nocturnal frontal lobe epilepsy. Clin Neurophysiol 111(Suppl 2):S129–S135, 2000.

15. RESTLESS LEGS SYNDROME AND PERIODIC LIMB MOVEMENT DISORDER

Suzanne Stevens, MD

RESTLESS LEGS SYNDROME

Epidemiology

1. What is the prevalence of restless legs syndrome?

Restless legs syndrome (RLS) is thought to be quite common as a result of epidemiologic studies done to determine prevalence. Estimates of prevalence in the general population range from 5% to 15%, although prevalence increases with age.

2. Who is at risk for secondary restless legs syndrome?

In idiopathic RLS no underlying disease causes the symptoms. Secondary RLS is coexistent with a disease thought to cause the RLS. Reasons for secondary RLS include renal disease, iron deficiency anemia, pregnancy, and peripheral neuropathy. Another cause for secondary RLS is provocation or exacerbations by antidepressant medication or medications resulting in blockade of the dopaminergic system. Medications reported to worsen RLS include metoclopramide, selective sertoninin reuptake inhibitors (SSRIs), tricyclic antidepressants, and antipsychotic medications such as haloperidol.

3. How common is restless legs syndrome in patients with renal failure?

RLS has been reported in 20% to 62% of patients undergoing dialysis. This patient group probably has the highest rate of secondary RLS.

4. How common is restless legs syndrome in other medical diseases?

The prevalence varies significantly according to different studies. Most studies report 20% prevalence in pregnancy, 5% prevalence in polyneuropathy, and 31% prevalence in patients with fibromyalgia.

5. What is the mean age of diagnosis of restless legs syndrome?

The mean age of diagnosis ranges from 27 to 41 years. Patients who present at a younger age (< 45 years old or early-onset RLS) are more likely to have a family history of RLS, typically progress more slowly, and are less likely to have ferritin abnormalities than those who present later (> 45 years old or late-onset RLS). In addition, patients presenting with late-onset RLS are more likely to have abnormalities on electromyography (EMG) consistent with small fiber neuropathy. Other characteristics of early-onset vs. late-onset RLS are shown in the table below.

Characteristics of Early-onset vs. Late-onset Restless Legs Syndrome

	Early Onset	Late Onset
Age of onset	< 45 years old	> 45 years old
Genetics	More likely familial	Less likely familial
Severity of symptoms	Less severe	More severe
Progression of RLS	Slower progression	Quicker progression
EMG findings	Usually normal	More likely to show changes of small fiber neuropathy
Ferritin levels	Usually normal	Often decreased

Pathophysiology

6. What part of the central nervous system is thought to be involved in the development of restless legs syndrome?

The dopaminergic system is thought to be the part of the central nervous system involved in developing RLS. This line of thought developed many years ago when a levodopa/carbidopa preparation was found to treat the symptoms of RLS, and even today dopaminergic compounds continue to be the first line of treatment. Additional evidence supporting the dopamineric system in RLS is that medications blocking the dopaminergic system (such as most antipsychotics and metoclopramide) exacerbate the symptoms of RLS. Furthermore, iron supplement improves RLS symptoms in certain populations of patients. Iron is a necessary cofactor for the rate-limiting step in dopamine synthesis (for the enzyme tyrosine hydroxylase). Low ferritin levels (< 50 μg/dl), even with normal complete blood count and iron levels, have been associated with RLS and in such patients iron supplement improves the symptoms of RLS. Ferritin reflects the body iron stores.

Ferritin and transferrin levels have been measured in the cerebrospinal fluid (CSF) of patients with RLS and compared with levels in controls. Although serum levels of ferritin and transferrin did not differ significantly between patients with RLS and controls, the CSF levels of ferritin were very low in patients with RLS compared with controls, and transferrin (which increases in iron-deficient states) increased in the CSF of patients with RLS compared with controls.

7. What do neuroimaging studies show in patients with restless legs syndrome?

Positron emission tomography (PET) and single-photon emission computed tomography (SPECT) studies have found mild decreases in striatal measurement of dopamine in patients with RLS vs. controls. In addition, dopamine-2 receptors are decreased in the basal ganglia of patients with RLS by SPECT studies. Magnetic resonance imaging (MRI) studies measuring iron in the brain have shown significantly reduced iron concentrations in the substantia nigra and putamen. It is unknown whether this finding is a cause or a result of dopaminergic deficiency in these regions. Functional magnetic resonance imaging (fMRI) was performed in 19 patients with RLS while they were experiencnig symptoms of discomfort. During sensory discomfort, fMRI showed activation of the bilateral cerebellum and contralateral thalamus. When periodic leg movements (PLMs) occurred, other brainstem structures were activated, including the red nuclei and reticular formation, which were not activated on voluntarily recreation of the PLM movement.

8. Discuss the circadian variation in the symptoms of restless leg movements.

Symptoms are typically worse in the evening, thus interfering with the ability to initiate sleep easily. Symptoms can persist through the night, causing fragmented nighttime sleep. Recordings of symptoms at different times throughout the 24-hour day with the suggested immobilization test (SIT) show that peak times for symptoms are between midnight and 2 AM, with a nadir for symptoms of between 9 AM and 1 PM. In these subjects, other aspects of their circadian rhythm, including temperature curves and cortisol levels, were normal. Of interest, dopamine and iron also have a circadian pattern with levels being lower at nighttime, when symptoms are worse.

9. What are the genetics behind restless legs syndrome?

A positive family history of RLS can be elicited in 40–50% of cases. First-degree relatives seem to be afflicted more often, following an autosomal dominant pattern of inheritance. A major susceptibility locus has been found on chromosome 12q. When inherited, RLS seems to begin at an earlier age and have a slower pattern of progression of symptoms compared with cases without a familial component.

10. What medications are known to worsen restless legs syndrome?

Medications that block the dopaminergic system are known to worsen the symptoms of RLS. Examples include antipsychotic medications that use dopaminergic blockage as their mechanism and metoclopramide. Antidepressant medications also may cause or exacerbate RLS symptoms.

Diagnosis and Classification

11. How do patients present with restless legs syndrome?

Patients often present with difficult in initiating and maintaining sleep due to the discomfort associated with RLS. Patients often describe their discomfort as being more prominent in the evening time, but symptoms may also occur during periods of relative immobility during the day-time as well, such as long plane rides, long-distance driving, and sitting during meetings or in the theater. These daytime symptoms may require treatment during the daytime hours, often on as-needed basis. Movement typically alleviates the discomfort, but symptoms return once the movement is stopped, giving the patient the appearance of being "restless."

During the night, patients try frequent position changes and even get out of bed to march in place at the bedside or simply walk around to relieve the pain (hence the name for the patient support group, the Nightwalkers). Typically, the more uncomfortable the position, the less prominent the RLS symptoms. Some patients choose to sleep on the floor to improve their symptoms. If the patient with RLS has periodic limb movement disorder as well (as 70–80% do), sleep may be fragmented by PLMs, causing electroencephalographic (EEG) arousals or frank awakenings; the bed partner may report kicking movements during sleep.

12. How do patients describe restless legs syndrome?

The descriptions of RLS include creepy-crawly sensation, burning, tingling, numbness, and Pepsi-Cola in the veins. Many patients use the word "indescribable."

13. How is restless leg syndrome diagnosed?

According to the International Restless Legs Syndrome Study Group, the diagnostic criteria for diagnosing RLS are as follows:
1. Focal akathisia usually with dysesthesias
    a. Irresistible desires or urges to move the legs
    b. Periodic episodes of distressing abnormal sensations in legs
2. Provocation of discomfort by rest
3. Relief of discomfort with activity
4. Circadian pattern showing a worsening of symptoms in the evening

14. What subjective scales have been validated to diagnose restless legs syndrome?

Two scales have been developed
- Johns Hopkins RLS Severity Scale (JHRLSS) uses a scale from 0 to 3, with 0 representing no symptoms, 1 for nighttime symptoms, 2 for evening symptoms and 3 for symptoms before 6 PM.
- International Restless Legs Syndrome Study Group (IRLSSG) severity scale has 10 items with each rated from 0 to 4.

15. Are any objective tests available to diagnose restless legs syndrome?

The suggested immobilization test (SIT) was developed to help diagnose RLS, but it still relies on the patient's subjective report of symptoms. The patient sits on a bed in an upright position and is instructed to hit a button when the uncomfortable sensations occur. This test is done for 20-60 minutes, and results are reported as an "index" of how many uncomfortable sensations are reported per hour. In addition, movements of the legs, called periodic leg movements of wakefulness (PLMW), are monitored and reported as an index.

16. What are polysomnographic features of restless legs syndrome?

Polysomnography (PSG) may show a long sleep onset latency and frequent awakenings. There may be frequent movements as the patient tries to find a comfortable position. Periodic limb movements of sleep (PLMS) may be seen in up to 80% of patients with RLS.

17. Can restless legs syndrome ever affect the arms?

Yes. The arms may be involved as well as the torso and abdomen. In one report, 48.7% of patients with RLS report symptoms in their arms. There are no reports of symptoms involving the head or neck.

18. What is the differential diagnosis of restless legs syndrome?

Akathisia, painful legs and moving toes, sleep starts, painful conditions, nocturnal leg cramps, arthritis, and polyneuropathy.

19. What is entailed in the evaluation of a patient with RLS?

Questions about medical conditions that can cause secondary RLS should be asked, including history of renal disease, peripheral neuropathy, iron deficiency, and pregnancy. Tests for ferritin levels and percentage of transferritin saturation should be ordered since results can be abnormal in both primary and secondary forms of RLS.

Prognosis and Treatment

20. How is restless legs syndrome treated?

Removal of precipitating or exacerbating medications should be done if possible. Checking ferritin level and percentage transferritin saturation with serum blood work should be done to see if the patient is a candidate for iron therapy.

21. How is secondary restless legs syndrome treated?

If possible, remove precipitating or exacerbating medications. If RLS is due to iron deficiency, treatment with an iron supplement many improve symptoms. When RLS occurs during pregnancy, the symptoms improve after delivery; however, if needed, pharmacotherapy can be instituted. Opioids are relatively safe for as-needed use in pregnancy, and pergolide, a dopaminergic medication, is in category B. RLS secondary to renal failure improves after transplantation but does not improve with dialysis. In other conditions causing secondary RLS, pharmacologic treatments described in question 22 may be of benefit.

22. What classes of drugs are used for treatment of restless legs syndrome?

Classes of medications used to treat RLS include dopamine precursors (levodopa), dopamnergic agonist medications, benzodiazepines, antiepileptic medication, opioids, and iron (if indicated by ferritin level).

Medications for Treatment of Restless Legs Syndrome

CLASS	NAME	STARTING DOSE	PEAK CONCENTRATION	HALF-LIFE
Dopamine agonists	Pramipexole	0.125 mg	2 hr	8–12 hr
	Pergolide*	0.05 mg		16 hr
	Ropinerole	0.25 mg	1–2 hr	6 hr
Dopamine precursor	Levodopa†	100 mg		1.5 hr
Benzodiazepines	Clonazepam	0.25 mg	1–4 hr	30–40 hr
	Triazolam	0.125 mg	2 hr	1.5–5.0 hr
	Temazepam	15 mg	30 min	8–15 hr
Opioids	Codeine	30 mg		2.5–3 hr
	Propoxyphene	100 mg	2–2.5 hr	6–12 hr
	Hydrocodone	5 mg	1.3 hr	4 hr
Antiepileptic	Gabapentin*	100 mg		5–7 hr

Table continued on next page

Medications for Treatment of Restless Legs Syndrome (continued)

CLASS	NAME	STARTING DOSE	PEAK CONCENTRATION	HALF-LIFE
Iron	Various formulations	325 mg (60-65 mg elemental iron)	Depends on formulation	

* Excreted renally.
† Usually given with carbidopa to decrease nausea.

23. What is the first-line treatment for restless legs syndrome?
The first-line treatment of RLS is dopaminergic agonist medication, such as pramipexole, pergolide, and ropinerole. The dopamine precursor levodopa combined with carbidopa has been used as well.

24. What difficulties may occur when dopaminergic medications are used to treat restless legs syndrome?
The dopaminergic medications have been associated with two phenomena called augmentation and rebound. **Augmentation** occurs when symptoms begin earlier in the day once dopaminergic medications are used in the evening. This problem can be helped by adding an additional dose of medication when the symptoms start, or a new medication may need to be tried. **Rebound** occurs when symptoms return in the middle of the night, usually with the short-acting preparation of carbidopa/levodopa. This problem may improve with a change to the longer-acting preparation.

25. How do benzodiazepines help in the treatment of restless legs syndrome? What are their side effects?
Clonazepam and triazolam, among others, can help with sleep initiation and consolidation. Although these medications have some muscle-relaxant properties, the main mechanism of action is thought to be increasing the brain's arousal threshold, allowing more consolidated, restful sleep. Side effects, such as daytime sedation with clonazepam, must be monitored.

26. For what type of symptoms might antiepileptic medications and opioids be most helpful?
Antiepileptic medications such as gabapentin and carbamazepine can be effective in the treatment of RLS, particularly if a painful component is present. Opioid medication is also particularly effective for treatment of a painful component.

27. When is iron indicated for treatment of restless legs syndrome?
If the ferritin level is below 50 μg/dl, treatment with supplemental iron may improve symptoms. The recommended dose of iron starts at 325 mg daily (ideally with an elemental iron content of 60–65 mg), which can be taken with vitamin C to facilitate absorption. This dose can be given up to 3 times daily with the goal of raising the ferritin to greater than 50 μg/dl, typically rechecking it every 3 months. Gastrointestinal side effects may limit dosing of iron. Intravenous iron therapy has been tried successfully in some patients.

PERIODIC LIMB MOVEMENT DISORDER

Epidemiology

28. What is the prevalence of periodic limb movement disorder?
Periodic limb movement disorder (PLMD) is more common with advancing age and is seen in up to 44% of people older than 65 years. PLMS (periodic limb movements of sleep) is also seen as an incidental finding in up to 5% of subjects.

Pathophysiology

29. Describe the clinical presentation of a patient with periodic limb movement disorder.

The presentation may be insomnia or hypersomnia. Witnessed nocturnal leg movements by someone may precipitate the visit.

30. What percentage of patients with periodic limb movement disorder have restless legs syndrome?

From 20% to 30% of patients with PLMD have RLS.

31. What is the effect of antidepressant medications on periodic limb movement disorder?

Antidepressant medication may worsen PLMD.

32. Which part of the neuraxis has been implicated in causing periodic limb movements of sleep?

Given that the periodic limb movements of sleep (PLMS) are similar to the Babinski sign seen in association with pyramindal tract disease (and in normal subjects during non-rapid-eye-movement [NREM] sleep), PLMS may represent an exaggerated disinhibition of motor activity. More specifically, PLMS may be an exaggerated response to suppression of supraspinal inhibitory forces during sleep. Neurophysiologic studies are consistent with the hypothesis of dis-inhibition at the level of brainstem (as seen in imaging studies discussed above) and spinal cord. Clinically, patients with spinal cord transections may develop PLMS, indicating that a generator may be located in the spinal cord.

Diagnosis and Classification

33. What are periodic limb movements?

Periodic limb movements (PLMs) are stereotyped movements of the extremities, occurring approximately every 20–40 seconds, usually during sleep. PLMs typically involve the legs but can involve the arms as well. The typical movement of the leg during sleep is similar to the triple-flexion response in that the movements include extension of the big toe with dorsiflexion of the ankle and sometimes even flexion of the knee and hip.

34. What is the difference between periodic limb movement disorder and periodic limb movements of sleep?

PLMD is a clinical diagnosis of the polysomnographic finding of PLMs coupled with the symptoms of insomnia or excessive daytime sleepiness. PLMS is a polysomnographic diagnosis.

35. How do patients with periodic limb movement disorder present?

Patients present with difficulty in initiating and maintaining sleep and may have daytime sleepiness. However, no objective studies have proved that PLMD can lead to daytime sleepiness, as measured by the multiple sleep latency test (MSLT). Twenty percent to 30% of patients with PLMD also have symptoms of RLS.

36. Can periodic limb movements be present during wakefulness?

Yes. Patients can report myoclonic movement during rest throughout the day. These are called periodic leg movements of wakefulness (PLMW).

37. How is periodic limb movement disorder diagnosed?

Polysomnography (PSG) is used for the diagnosis of PLMD. The activity of the anterior tibialis muscle is monitored by electromyogram (EMG). PLMs are reported by a PLM index, indicating the number of movements recorded per hour of sleep, with a value > 5 being abnormal. PLMs are more commonly noted during NREM sleep and are more rare during REM sleep, although they may occur primarily in REM sleep with other disorders such as REM without atonia or REM sleep behavior disorder.

38. How do periodic limb movements appear during a PSG recording?

They appear as periodic increases in EMG activity of the anterior tibialis muscle of the lower extremities. They may occur with or without secondary arousals. A sample PSG epoch showing PLMs is shown in Figure 1.

39. How are periodic limb movements scored?

PLMs are scored using Coleman's criteria. To be classified as PLMs, each movement must be from 0.5 to 5 seconds in length, be separated by 4–90 seconds, and occur in a train of 4 movements.

40. How are periodic limb movements reported on a PSG result?

The PLMs are reported as an index, indicating the number of movements averaged per hour of sleep. Often they are further classified into periodic limb movements with arousal. In general, a periodic leg movement index < 5 is normal. An index of 5–20 indicates a mild disorder; an index of 20–40, moderate disorder; and an index > 40, severe disorder.

41. Can actigraphy contribute to the diagnosis of periodic limb movement disorder?

Actigraphy has potential to be used for diagnosis and follow-up of PLMD. However, it has yet to be validated in studies with large numbers of patients.

42. What is the differential diagnosis of periodic limb movement disorder?

Hypnic myoclonus, phasic REM twitches, propriospinal myoclonus, and seizure.

43. How often are periodic limb movements of sleep associated with other sleep disorders?

PLMS are seen often in narcolepsy (up to two-thirds of patients), and their prevalence in narcoleptics increases with age. PLMS are seen in up to 70% of patients with REM sleep behavior disorder and are often seen in patents with obstructive sleep apnea. As stated previously, 80% of patients with RLS have PLMS on PSG. Of interest, evidence suggests that RLS, narcolepsy, and REM sleep behavior disorder may be due to dopamine deficiency, and they improve with stimulation of the dopaminergic pathways, indicating a possible contribution of dopamine deficiency to PLMS as well.

44. What coexisting medical conditions can be associated with periodic limb movements of sleep?

Anemia, renal failure, peripheral neuropathy, and rheumatoid arthritis are associated with PLMD (as with RLS). In addition, PLMS have been seen in children with attention deficit-hyperactivity disorder as well as patients with Tourette's syndrome.

Prognosis and Treatment

45. What is the effect on periodic limb movement disorder when sleep-disordered breathing is treated with continuous positive airway pressure?

PLMD may improve, remain unchanged or become more severe when sleep-disordered breathing is treated with continuous positive airway pressure (CPAP). If the baseline study showed respiratory effort-related arousals (RERAs), which can be incorrectly scored as PLMS, these may dramatically improve with CPAP.

46. What are the pharmacologic treatments for periodic leg movement disorder?

The treatment for PLMD is similar to that for RLS (see question 22). The first-line treatment is a dopaminergic agonist, such as pramipexole, pergolide, and ropinerole. Bromocriptine has

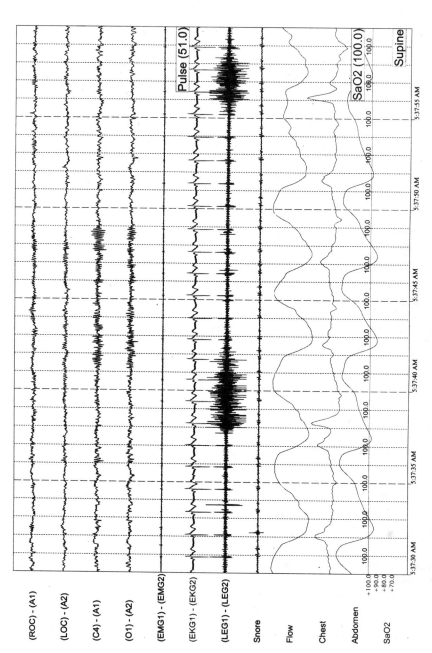

Figure 1. A typical example of periodic limb movements. Two separate limb movements are shown on this 30-second epoch with an associated arousal on the first limb movement.

been used as well. The dopamine precursor levodopa has been shown to be effective. Other treatment options include benzodiazepines, antiepileptic medications, and opioids. No studies have evaluated the role of iron therapy in patients with PLMD.

BIBLIOGRAPHY

1. Allen RP, Earley CJ: Restless legs syndrome: A review of clinical and pathophysiologic features. J Clin Neurophysiol 18(2):128–147, 2001.
2. Allen RP, Picchietti D, Hening WA, et al: Restless legs syndrome: Diagnostic criteria, special considerations, and epidemiology. A report from the Restless Legs Syndrome Diagnosis and Epidemiology Workshop at the National Institutes of Health. Sleep Med 4:101–119, 2003.
3. Chesson AL, Jr, et al: AASM Standards of Practice Committee. Practice parameters for the treatment of restless legs syndrome and periodic limb movement disorder. An American Academy of Sleep Medicine Report. Sleep;22:961–968, 1999.
4. Earley CJ: Restless legs syndrome. N Engl J Med 348:2103–2109, 2003.
5. Early CJ, Connor JR, Beard JL, et al: Abnormalities in CSF concentrations of ferritin and transferring in restless legs syndrome. Neurology 54:1698–1700, 2000.
6. Hening W, Allen R, Earley C, et al: The treatment of restless legs syndrome and periodic limb movement disorder: An American Academy of Sleep Medicine Review. Sleep 22:970–999, 1999.

16. DREAMING

Rosalind Cartwright, PhD

1. Define dreaming.

Dreaming refers to the internally generated perceptual experiences that occur during sleep and are accepted by the dreamer at the time as reality. Dreams are predominantly visual but may include other senses as well. In fact, they are hallucinations, which, if experienced during the waking state, might be considered "psychotic."

2. How frequently do humans dream?

All humans have the brain state conditions that support dream experience on a cyclic basis—approximately every 90 minutes of the major sleep period. There are 3–5 such episodes in a 7- to 8-hour sleep night, each lasting a little longer than the previous one. Dreams typically occupy about 20% of the sleep time of adults.

3. Since dreaming takes place during sleep, how can it be studied objectively?

Dreaming is investigated by identifying the presence of the brain state known as rapid-eye-movement (REM) sleep. This state is marked by three components: a sleep electroencephalographic (EEG) recording showing low-voltage, high-frequency brain waves, indicating high brain activation; a drop of the muscle tone from the chin area, as recorded on electromyography (EMG); and the presence of rapid saccadic movements of the eyes, as recorded on electro-oculography (EOG). When awakened abruptly during this state, sleepers are able to report the dream experience on about 85% of occasions. In other words, of the 3–5 episodes of REM sleep during a typical night for a normal adult, three or four yield a report of ongoing perceptual experience. These reports are captured on audiotape for later analysis. This approach yields much more dream data than can be obtained from spontaneous (unaided) morning recall.

4. Do animals dream?

All mammals have cycles of REM sleep. Although language is required to report a dream, it has been inferred that monkeys have visual experiences during REM sleep from experiments carried out in conjunction with the space program. Monkeys who were rewarded for making correct visual discriminations between symbols displayed on a screen during daytime training sessions were observed making the same behavioral response during REM sleep, suggesting they were "seeing things" at that time. Many pet owners have also noted that their dog or cat goes through periods when the eyes appear to be moving rapidly under the lids while they whine or make small twitching movements as if engaged in an imaginary chase.

5. Are there natural developmental changes in the amount of dreaming?

REM sleep is highly prominent in neonates, making up about 50% of their sleep. This activated brain state appears to be correlated with the development of synaptic connections in the brain since the percentage of this sleep drops at about 1 year of age to half the initial amount. At what age REM sleep becomes associated with the experience of dreaming, as we know it, is hard to say until language develops. However, in a classic study of children's dreams Foulkes (1982) showed a close parallel between the cognitive level of the child in waking and the cognitive level displayed in dream reports. The first reports of young children aged 3–5 years are of a single image, predominantly of animals, such as "a dog barking" or a "frog in the water." By ages 9 to 10, the same children display much more narrative complexity in their dream reports in keeping with their waking level of cognitive development.

6. Do men and women differ in their dreams?

Studies of differences in the dreams of the two genders have shown remarkable stability in the face of major social changes toward more gender equality in waking experience. Differences between the dreams of men and women studied in 1950 and 1980 reported that men have more outdoor settings in their dreams, whereas the dreams of women were more often set in an interior location. Men had more hostile and aggressive interactions in their dreams, whereas women had more friendly interactions. Men had a predominance of male characters, whereas women had a more nearly equal ratio of male and female characters (Hall, Domhoff, Blick, Wesner, 1982).

7. Does the nature of the dream content change with aging?

Dreams appear to reflect waking emotional concerns; therefore, it is not surprising to find that the elderly have more dreams of the past and more dreams concerning physical health and death than middle-aged people.

8. Why do some people remember their dreams often, whereas others have little or no spontaneous recall?

Recall of dreams varies widely from person to person. Some people regularly recall one or more dreams on morning awakening, whereas others claim that they "never dream." Typically women report more frequent recall than men. This finding appears to be related to the finding that women are more aware of and responsive to their inner emotions during waking, whereas men are more focused on external information.

High among the variables accounting for the differences in recall of dreams are motivation, depth of sleep, verbal skills, and personality. Motivation to recall is probably the most powerful of these factors. The same factors that govern what is remembered from waking experience appear also to contribute to memory for dreams—namely, the degree of interest in and importance to the individual of the information. Failure to recall dreams does not carry the same penalty as failure to remember one's Social Security number or what the boss asked us to do. Even people with poor recall of dreams who enter psychotherapy have a dramatic increase in their memory for dreams if the therapist requires that dreams be reported during each session. Light sleepers find it easier to recall their dreams than people who sleep deeply. People who sleep more lightly are closer to waking throughout sleep, and brief arousal into a waking state appears to be necessary to fix dream experiences into memory. People who are more anxious, either chronically or acutely, may also sleep more lightly and have higher spontaneous recall of their dreams than people without anxiety.

9. What are some of the difficulties in understanding the meaning of dreams?

There are different theories suggesting reasons why the meaning of dreams is not straightforward. One proposed by Crick and Mitchison (1983) is that dreams have no meaning. The images of REM represent only random impressions from the previous day as they are expunged from memory by the high activation of the REM sleep state. Older theoretic positions based on Freud's *Interpretation of Dreams* (1938) hold that dream meaning is disguised to allow the expression of unacceptable wishes during the safety of a sleep state when there is no threat of action due to the accompanying loss of muscle tone. Current dream research supports the view that the meaning of dreams that are spontaneously recalled at home presents a particular difficulty because usually only the last dream of the night is recalled. The meaning may be hard to decipher because it is out of the context of the several dreams that preceded it. An analogy is trying to understand a novel by reading only the last chapter.

Other constraints on understanding dreams come from the difficulty posed by the need for dreamers to translate their original visual experience into a verbal report. This skill is not highly practiced in our culture. Those who are motivated to understand their dreams can increase their ability by practice; they may keep a dream diary for a few weeks and review it in relation to their ongoing waking concerns. Repetitive patterns are soon observed and cue the dreamer to the emotional meanings of the perceptual images.

10. Do dreams reveal an unknown aspect of ourselves, or are they simply our usual thoughts expressed in "picture language"?

There is some agreement among those who have conducted research on dreams, collected from REM periods, in subjects whose personality and current waking concerns have also been well studied. The major differences between conscious waking thoughts and dreams lie in the difference of the thought style of the two states. During waking the predominant style is linear, based on logical connections, whereas in REM the style is more global, following emotional connections. For those who are well tuned to the emotional implications of their daily experience, dreams appear to illustrate their present state of mind rather well. However, those who are rather unaware of their own emotional responses on an ongoing basis find their dreams to be foreign to them.

11. Are dreams the source of creative solutions to problems?

The style of thinking about problems in waking and dreaming differs. The waking style is more convergent, whereas dreaming is more divergent. It is not surprising, therefore, that different solutions may be reached to the same problem. Whether the solutions from one state are "better" than those from the other is debatable. Clear, well-controlled research is difficult to carry out on this topic. The data in support of more creative resolutions following a dream are mostly anecdotal but so common that this question must remain open for exploration in future studies.

12. What happens if dreaming is suppressed by medication or limited by lack of sufficient sleep?

One of the first attempts to understand the function of REM sleep was carried out by waking sleepers whenever the first signs of REM sleep appeared and keeping them from returning to sleep for 3–5 minutes (Dement, 1960). This landmark study showed that when REM is not permitted to occur over three or more nights, the percentage of REM sleep show a dramatic increase on the next night of uninterrupted sleep. This finding was interpreted at the time as proving a "need" to dream.

Although there has been some refinement of this conclusion based on subsequent work with other populations, the rule of thumb still holds that REM sleep shows a rebound following the lifting of any condition that has reduced its normal proportion of sleep. Whether this finding proves a "need" to dream is another question. The answer depends on designing studies that will test specific psychological functions of dream experience. The evidence at this time is sparse. One of the psychological hypotheses being tested is that dreaming aids retention of new learning. The proof would be if the content of dreams after learning some new task showed elements associating the new learning with previous related experiences already in long-term memory and, if so, retention was higher on the next day. This work has been reviewed recently by De Konick (2000).

13. How does a nightmare differ from a dream?

A nightmare is defined as a dream that is frightening enough to awaken the sleeper. Although nightmares are common in children, they tend to reduce in frequency as children grow in competence and have less anxiety about handling themselves in their waking lives. Nightmares increase in frequency after stressful events and are a hallmark symptom of posttraumatic stress disorder (PTSD). They are also more frequent during a period of increased REM sleep following withdrawal from REM-suppressing medications, such as the tricyclic antidepressants, or the introduction of continuous positive airway pressure (CPAP) for the treatment of severe sleep apnea. If nightmares persist, they can be treated by application of the principles of cognitive behavioral therapy to the dream experience (Cartwright and Lamberg, 2000),

14. How does a night terror differ from a nightmare?

The term *night terror* refers to a non-REM phenomenon while a nightmare occurs during REM sleep. The night terror occurs most often in young children, within the first hour of sleep before the first REM period of the night. Behaviorally, the child sits up in bed abruptly, screams as if frightened, and has glazed eyes and an increased heart rate. However, no dream content is reported, and the child typically has no recall of the episode next morning. Night terror is one of a family of sleep disorders called the parasomnias, which include sleepwalking and nocturnal enuresis. They occur in about 15% of prepubescent children. They run in families with the prevalence doubling when both parents were affected as children. Night terrors gradually reduce in frequency during adolescence. They are disorders of arousal and are not dreams.

15. Is a sleepwalker acting out his or her dreams?

No. As with night terrors, most childhood sleepwalkers are aroused early in their first or second cycle of non-REM sleep before dreaming has taken place. The one exception is the elderly person suffering from some neurologic insult or degenerative disorder that interferes with the loss of muscle tone during REM sleep. Such patients may suffer from REM behavior disorder, which allows a motor response to the ongoing dream scenario. Most cases of both REM behavior disorder and sleepwalking can be controlled by small doses of clonazepam, a benzodiazapine with a muscle-relaxing component.

16. Are differences in dreaming associated with different medical conditions?

The evidence from formal studies is small but intriguing. One classic study focused on a small group of patients whose dreams were recorded from each REM period for several nights before and after surgery. The dreams showed fears of the invasive procedure before surgery, followed by a more positive outlook afterward. Perhaps the most convincing study was of cardiology patients whose dreams of death or separation from loved ones were correlated with ejection fraction data. Patients reporting no dreams had the most severe disease according to ejection fraction results. Men with severe disease dreamed most often of death, whereas women with severe disease dreamed more often of separation from loved ones. Some have suggested that dreams may foretell the appearance of a disease before waking symptoms are noted.

17. Do congenitally blind dream?

People who have never had sight do have REM periods, although their eye movements are greatly reduced in amplitude. Their dreams are more often constructed from the senses that they use in waking to construct their maps of reality: sounds, textures, and kinesthetic experiences. These senses form the basis of their dream fantasies.

18. What are the current theories of dream function?

Theories of dream function fall into two categories: those based on recalled dreams and those based on sleep laboratory data. The first category is limited to dreams that are spontaneously remembered, most often by people who are in some emotional difficulty. These theories tend to emphasize the role of dreams in revealing unrecognized connections between present feelings and past experiences. They hypothesize that waking emotion instigates the selection of older memory material for the illustration of how the present relates to the past. Theories derived from laboratory-collected dreams are based on a wider sample of the nightly data and more often have a forward thrust, hypothesizing that the ways in which several dreams within one night relate to each other have differing effects on the subsequent waking state of mind. This is called the mood-regulatory theory of dreaming.

19. Do brain imaging studies help the understanding of dreaming?

The ability to study the areas of the brain that are more active during REM sleep than during non-REM sleep and/or waking have given a substantial impetus to such work. Positron emission tomographic (PET) studies conducted on sleeping subjects reveal a higher level of activity in the amygdala and paralimbic system during REM sleep, implicating involvement of the long-term emotional memory system.

20. Would we be better off if we could remember our dreams?

Given that dreaming appears to be a universal human activity with a high degree of regularity and similarity to other rhythmic systems and that recall appears to vary with the degree of light or disrupted sleep, it seems that it is not necessary to recall dreams for them to carry out their putative function. Perhaps the best rule of thumb may be that when dreams disrupt sleep they may indicate a malfunction of emotional information processing that requires some attention. Dreams may be a source of interest for people in the arts or people motivated to achieve a higher degree of self-awareness who are not in a state of maladjustment. Such people can learn to increase their level of recall with minimal effort by following certain simple tips.

21. How can the memory of dreams be trained?

1. Choose a night when sleep will not be interrupted by an alarm clock in the morning—preferably a week-end night when sleep can be terminated naturally. This step ensures that the awakening will be from REM sleep or close to it since REM predominates at the end of the night.
2. Increase the intention to remember by setting the stage with pad and pencil handy or a voice-activated tape recorder at the bedside.
3. Prolong the transition period from REM to waking by keeping the eyes closed and remaining still while mentally rehearsing the last dream. Once these images are firmly in mind, give the dream a title. A verbal cue prompts the memory to recall the scenario. Then write or record all that you can remember.

22. Can a dream be changed by the dreamer?

For the most part dreams appear to have a life of their own, beyond the dreamer's control. Some people have the ability to observe that they are dreaming. This ability is called "lucid dreaming." People with this ability can learn to change the course of an ongoing dream. This skill is not common, but it may help to learn to control nightmares or other disturbing dream scenarios.

23. What causes people to dream as soon as their head hits the pillow?

Several conditions may be responsible for this experience.

- The person may be experiencing a normal transition from waking to stage 1 sleep when thoughts are often experienced as single images, usually without the narrative continuity of dreaming.
- The person may be having a real REM sleep episode complete with a dream intrusion into sleep onset. This event, called a hypnagogic hallucination, is due to a sleep disorder called narcolepsy. Such people have other signs of the disorder, including excessive daytime sleepiness.
- The person may have a sleep-onset REM period as the result of a very disrupted sleep schedule in which the timing of the usual 90-minute cycles has been upset over a period of time.
- The person may have a REM-onset episode due to the rebound of REM sleep after release from some condition that suppressed REM over a period of several days or more.

24. Are certain dreams common to many people?

To the extent that all humans share some common experiences, a few types of dreams are reported by many people:

- Dreams of falling or flying
- Dreams of physical danger from others (e.g., being chased or stalked by animals or persons with evil intent)
- Dreams of social embarrassment or glory
- Dreams of being lost or late (e.g., missing the train, boat, or plane)
- Dreams of being unprepared to cope with some expectation (e.g., examinations)

These dreams reflect anxieties, or their opposites, commonly encountered in learning the physical laws, social rules, and standards by which we judge our own behavior.

25. Where do the images and other perceptions that make up dreams come from?

Clearly they come from within, from bits stored in memory and stimulated to replay in response to reminders encountered in waking. The strangeness of dreams comes from the juxtaposition of combinations of images according to a thread of emotional connection often not recognized or understandable to the waking mind.

26. Why do we sometimes have the same dream over and over?

Dreams rarely repeat exactly but do repeat in theme. Presumably they represent an issue of continuing emotional concern.

27. Do dreams represent an underutilized resource of the mind?

This question is hard to address with good methodology. Most families can report some incident in which a relative had a dream of a forthcoming event, a death or accident, that occured shortly afterward. Whether the mind in sleep has the ability to "tune in" to information not yet available in waking reality is a teasing prospect. However, no one keeps track of the many instances in which a dreamed event does not occur to test whether there are more correct predictions than would be expected by chance. The sleeping mind has not been thoroughly studied to see whether anything can be gained by "sleeping on" a decision beyond what benefit a period of rest provides. This theory awaits evidence from well-designed studies.

BIBLIOGRAPHY

1. Cartwright R, Lamberg L: Crisis Dreaming. ASJA Press, 2000.
2. Crick F, Mitchison G: The function of dream sleep. Nature 304:111–114, 1983.
3. De Konick J: Waking experiences and dreaming. In Kryger M, Roth T, Dement W (eds): Principles and Practice of Sleep Medicine, 3rd ed. Philadelphia, W.B. Saunders, 2000, pp 502–509.
4. Dement W: The effect of dream deprivation. Science 131:1705–1707, 1960.
5. Foulkes D: Children's Dreams: Longitudinal Studies. New York, John Wiley & Sons, 1982.
6. Freud S. The Interpretation of Dreams. In Brill A (ed): The Basic Writings of Sigmund Freud. Modern Library, New York, 1938, pp 181–549.
7. Hall C, Domhoff W, Blick K, Weesner K: The dreams of college men and women in 1950 and 1980: A comparison of dream contents and sex differences. Sleep 5:188–194, 1982.

III. Sleep and Other Medical Conditions

17. SLEEP AND CARDIOVASCULAR DISORDERS

Babak Mokhlesi, MD

PATHOPHYSIOLOGY

1. What happens to the cardiovascular system during normal sleep?

Normal non–rapid-eye-movement (NREM) sleep leads to a decline in heart rate, mean arterial pressure, and sympathetic nerve activity. REM sleep is associated with increased sympathetic activation leading to elevation in mean arterial pressure and heart rate that is close to the awake state. The majority of sleep is spent in non-REM; therefore, sleep represents a state of cardiovascular and autonomic quiescence leading to reduced myocardial workload.

2. What are the acute physiologic effects of obstructive apneas on the cardiovascular system?

An obstructive event is accompanied by a surge in heart rate, systemic blood pressure, and sympathetic nerve activity. In moderate-to-severe cases of sleep apnea-hypopnea syndrome (SAHS), the repetitive obstructive respiratory events counteract the normal state of cardiovascular quiescence. Three features of obstructive events give rise to the abnormal cardiovascular oscillations: increased negative intrathoracic pressure, more frequent arousals, and increased hypoxia. Exaggerated negative intrathoracic pressure is intended to overcome the upper airway obstruction. However, it can increase left ventricular afterload and venous return to the right ventricle, leading to its overdistention, which may impede left ventricular filling. Arousals and sleep fragmentation, independent of apnea, can cause an increase in sympathetic activation, leading to abrupt surges in heart rate and blood pressure.

3. Does intermittent nocturnal hypoxia contribute to development of systemic hypertension independently of apneas and arousals?

The role of hypoxia as a contributor to surges in blood pressure remains controversial. In animal models, there is a direct relationship between intermittent nocturnal hypoxia and development of hypertension. In humans, however, apneas with oxygen supplementation led to the same degree of postapneic elevation in blood pressure as hypoxic apneas. Furthermore, hypoxia without apneas or arousals was not associated with blood pressure elevations.

4. In addition to surges in catecholamines, what other circulating hormones or growth factors are increased in patients with SAHS?

Multiple hormones are elevated in SAHS, including renin, aldosterone, and vasopressin. All three hormones lead to vasopressor effects and fluid retention. Atrial natriuretic peptide is secreted in response to right atrial dilatation; its levels are elevated in proportion to the degree of hypoxia in SAHS. It promotes diuresis, natriuresis, and vasodilation. These effects may explain, in part, increased nocturia in patients with SAHS. Treatment with CPAP reduces nocturnal urinary atrial natriuretic peptide levels.

Recently, there has been an emerging interest in establishing the relationship between SAHS and elevation in serum levels of vascular endothelial growth factor. Whether this hypoxia-sensitive glycoprotein contributes to the long-term adaptation of sleep apnea syndrome to recurrent nocturnal hypoxia remains to be elucidated.

5. Does SAHS alter platelet aggregability, coagulability, and blood viscosity?

Yes. Several investigators have demonstrated that, compared with normal controls, patients with SAHS have increased platelet aggregability, increased blood viscosity, higher fibrinogen levels, and higher levels of factor VII. However, only a few studies have been able to demonstrate a positive effect of continuous positive airway pressure (CPAP) on the coagulation system.

6. Does the level of C-reactive protein increase in patients with SAHS?

Yes. Mounting evidence indicates that C-reactive protein is a strong predictor of cardiovascular disease. Two studies have shown a direct association between severity of SAHS and elevation in C-reactive protein, even after controlling for age, sex, and body mass index. Yokoe et al. demonstrated a significant drop in C-reactive protein after 1 month of CPAP therapy. The long-term clinical significance of improvement in C-reactive protein with CPAP therapy needs further investigation.

7. Does SAHS increase atherogenesis?

No direct evidence indicates that SAHS causes atherosclerosis. Nevertheless, increased oxidative stress, as evidenced by increased production of reactive oxygen species in neutrophils and monocytes, is seen in patients with OSA. Increased oxidative stress is associated with elevated levels of the three soluble circulating adhesion molecules: intracellular adhesion molecule-1 (ICAM-1), vascular cell adhesion molecule-1 (VCAM-1), and E-selectin. Conversely, treatment with CPAP can lower basal reactive oxygen species, downregulate adhesion molecule expression, and decrease leukocyte adherence to human endothelial cells in culture.

SAHS AND HYPERTENSION

8. Does SAHS increase the risk of developing systemic hypertension?

Yes. Two large prospective studies of middle-aged and older adults (Sleep Heart Health Study and the Wisconsin Sleep Cohort Study) have established, in a definitive manner, a positive association between SAHS and systemic hypertension. Both studies demonstrated an increased odds ratio for hypertension even after adjusting for confounding variables such as base-line hypertension, body habitus, and alcohol and cigarette use.

9. Is there a relationship between the severity of SAHS, as determined by the apnea-hypopnea index (AHI), and the risk of developing hypertension?

Yes. There is a dose-response association between severity of SAHS as measured by AHI and prevalence of hypertension. In the Wisconsin Sleep Cohort Study, the odds ratio for hypertension, after adjusting for confounding variables, increased from 1.42 in patients with an AHI between 0.1 and 4.9 to 2.89 in patients with an AHI ≥ 15. In other words, an AHI ≥ 15 increases the risk of developing hypertension by nearly three-fold.

10. What are the clinical implications of "nondipping" of nocturnal blood pressure?

The nocturnal blood pressure is on average 15% below daytime levels (i.e., dipping or dippers). The risk of cardiovascular complications is higher in nondippers. The phenomenon of dipping is preserved in most patients with essential hypertension, but many normotensive and hypertensive patients with SAHS are nondippers. Nondipping appears to be more prevalent in African Americans with SAHS. Effective CPAP therapy can convert patients with SAHS who are nondippers into dippers.

11. Does CPAP improve systemic blood pressure in hypertensive patients with SAHS?

Yes. CPAP can improve systemic blood pressure in hypertensive patients with SAHS. Initial randomized clinical trials that showed no effect or minimal effect of CPAP on blood pressure had not enrolled hypertensive patients. However, several nonrandomized trials and a recent randomized, placebo-controlled trial have shown that CPAP treatment leads to a substantial reduction in both daytime and nighttime arterial blood pressure in hypertensive patients with SAHS. All of these trials have documented an average drop of 10 mmHg in mean, systolic, and diastolic pressures. These results have significant clinical relevance since a 10-mmHg reduction in mean blood pressure leads to 37% reduction in coronary heart disease event risk and 56% reduction in stroke event risk.

12. Is the prevalence of SAHS higher in patients with refractory hypertension compared with nonrefractory hypertension?

Yes. The prevalence of SAHS is quite high in patients with refractory hypertension, defined as blood pressure above 140/90 mmHg while the patient is taking three or more sensible antihypertensive agents at maximum dose. In a cross-sectional, uncontrolled study of 41 patients with refractory hypertension enrolled from a university hypertension clinic, the prevalence of SAHS (AHI ≥ 10) was 83%. Most patients were obese with mean body mass index of 34. In contrast, a controlled study of nonrefractory hypertensives reported a prevalence of OSA (AHI ≥ 10) of 23%. These patients had a lower mean body mass index of approximately 29. In an uncontrolled study of 11 patients with refractory hypertension and SAHS, two months of CPAP reduced 24-hour systolic blood pressure by a mean of 11 mmHg.

SAHS AND CONGESTIVE HEART FAILURE

13. What is the prevalence of SAHS in patients with congestive heart failure (CHF)?

In a large retrospective study of patients with stable systolic heart failure, the prevalence of OSA (defined as AHI > 10) was 72%. The prevalence of central sleep apnea (CSA) was 33%. However, the prevalence of sleep-disordered breathing in this study may have been an overestimation due to selection bias. In a smaller prospective study, 51% of all patients had AHI > 10; 40% had CSA and 11% had SAHS.

14. Does SAHS increase the risk of CHF?

Yes. In the Sleep Heart Health Study, the presence of SAHS, defined as AHI > 11, was associated with a 2.38 relative odds ratio for self-reported CHF after adjusting for other known risk factors.

15. What are the key pathophysiologic mechanisms leading to Cheyne-Stokes respiration with central sleep apnea (CSR-CSA) in patients with systolic CHF?

Several potential mechanisms may lead to CSR-CSA in patients with CHF:

- Patients with CHF and CSR-CSA have lower partial pressure of carbon dioxide in arterial blood ($PaCO_2$) during wakefulness and sleep than patients with CHF who do not have CSR-CSA. Many of these patients have an enhanced sensitivity to CO_2 that may destabilize breathing during sleep. During sleep, the $PaCO_2$ rises by 3–6 mmHg, becoming the most potent stimulus of breathing. If the $PaCO_2$ decreases below the apneic threshold, breathing ceases. This state of CSA results in an increase in the $PaCO_2$, which in the presence of enhanced sensitivity to CO_2 can lead to hyperventilation. This response may in turn lower the $PaCO_2$ below the apneic threshold, causing periodic breathing with recurring cycles of apnea and hyperventilation.
- The role of hypoxia in CSR-CSA remains unclear, especially since these patients are not hypoxic while awake. However, hypoxia during apneas may exacerbate the ventilatory response to CO_2 at the end of apneas.
- Upper airway instability and collapse can increase ventilation excessively, leading to a central apnea.
- Prolonged circulation time between the lungs and the central chemoreceptors can destabilize respiratory control, contributing minimally to periodic breathing.

16. What is the impact of CSR-CSA in patients with systolic CHF?

Sleep-disordered breathing due to CSR-CSA can cause sleep fragmentation, increased sympathetic activity, excessive daytime sleepiness, and oscillations in heart rate and blood pressure. All of these changes can increase ventricular arrhythmias in patients with CHF and CSR-CSA. Moreover, CSR-CSA increases the chance of death or need for cardiac transplantation in patients with systolic CHF independently of other risk factors.

17. Does CPAP improve cardiac function in patients with CSR-CSA and systolic CHF?

Yes. CPAP decreases preload and left ventricular afterload in a failing heart and in patients with stable chronic systolic CHF. Long-term nocturnal CPAP increases left ventricular ejection fraction by approximately 8%. In a prospective, randomized, controlled trial, CPAP reduced mortality and cardiac transplantation in patients with systolic CHF and CSR-CSA.

18. How is nasal CPAP titrated in patients with CSR-CSA?

In the absence of obstructive apneas and/or hypopneas, CPAP is titrated to between 10 and 12.5 cmH$_2$O. Pressures above this level may exacerbate central apneas.

19. In addition to CPAP, what other treatments can improve CSR-CSA?

In addition to optimal management of CHF, nocturnal supplemental oxygen and theophylline have been shown to decrease CSR-CSA. However, they do not lead to an improvement in cardiac function. Moreover, long-term theophylline use may induce arrhythmogenecity.

20. How does SAHS exacerbate cardiac function in systolic CHF?

Obstructive apneas and hypopneas have a negative impact on the cardiac function in a failing heart. Negative intrathoracic pressure swings lead to (1) an increase in left ventricular afterload and (2) an increase in venous return to the right ventricle with overdistention and leftward shift of the interventricular septum, which further decrease left ventricular filling. Moreover, arousals lead to an increase in sympathetic vasoconstrictor outflow, which further increases left ventricular afterload. Hypoxia and hypercapnia decrease oxygen delivery to the stressed myocardium and cause transient pulmonary hypertension. SAHS may thus have an adverse effect in heart failure.

21. Discuss the role of CPAP in patients with SAHS and systolic CHF.

A recent controlled, randomized trial of CPAP in patients with stable systolic CHF and SAHS demonstrated a significant improvement in left ventricular systolic function and a 10-mmHg decrease in systolic blood pressure after only 1 month of CPAP use. The change in the left ventricular ejection fraction from baseline to 1 month was significantly greater in the group treated with CPAP than in the control group (8.8% vs. 1.5%).

SAHS AND CARDIAC ARRHYTHMIAS

22. Does sleep lead to increased arrhythmias in normal people?

No. The increased parasympathetic activity during sleep has a significant effect on cardiac electrophysiology, causing a decrease in heart rate, slowing of conduction in the atrioventricular (AV) node, and prolongation of cardiac refractory periods. These changes exert an antiarrhythmogenic effect during sleep.

23. What are the most common arrhythmias reported during sleep in normal people?

Sinus bradycardia and sinus arrhythmia are the most common arrhythmias reported in normal people during sleep. Figure 1 shows a typical sinus arrhythmia with heart-rate slowing after inspiration. Sinus pauses ≤ 2 seconds and second-degree atrioventricular heart block (Mobitz type I) have been reported in up to 30% and 6% of healthy people, respectively. The majority of studies in healthy people have shown an antiarrhythmic effect of sleep on premature ventricular contractions.

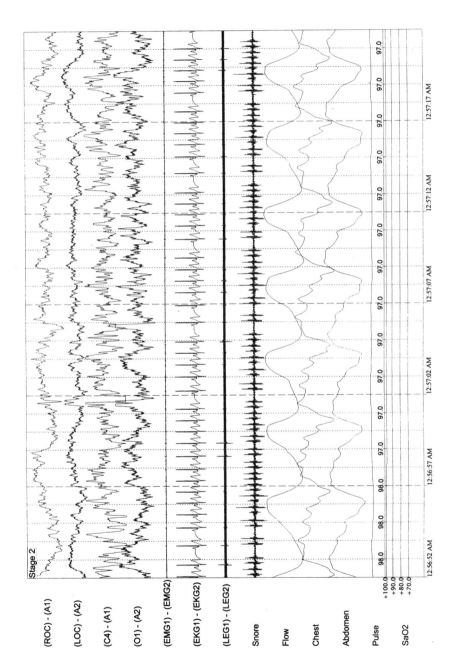

Figure 1. Typical sinus arrhythmia with slowing of heart rate after inspiration.

24. Does SAHS increase cardiac arrhythmias?

The relationship between SAHS and cardiac arrhythmias remains controversial. Two large studies have reported a prevalence of cardiac arrhythmias as high as 48% to 58% in patients with SAHS compared with nonapneic snorers. Several other studies have reported a much lower prevalence of arrhythmias that was not significantly different from that in nonapneic snorers.

25. What is the most common arrhythmia seen in patients with SAHS?

Bradycardia with or without alternating tachycardia is the most common arrhythmia observed during an apneic episode. The heart rate declines during an apneic episode, and once apnea is relieved, tachycardia ensues. Sinus arrest and atrioventricular block have been demonstrated in as many as 10% to 30% of patients with SAHS, and both occur more commonly during REM sleep. Figure 2 shows severe sinus bradycardia during polysomnography. Severity of SAHS and morbid obesity may be independent predictors of heart block. It remains controversial as to whether the severity of oxygen desaturation during an apneic episode correlates with cardiac arrhythmias or not. The overall clinical significance of the rhythm disturbances observed with SAHS remains to be elucidated. The prevalence of ventricular tachycardia has been reported to range between 3% and 13%. Ventricular premature beats are even more common and seem to be related to the severity of SAHS.

26. Does CPAP decrease cardiac arrhythmias in SAHS?

Yes. Several studies have reported a decrease in cardiac arrhythmias (including ventricular arrhythmias) in patients with SAHS after successful CPAP therapy or tracheostomy. Moreover, CPAP decreases ventricular irritability in patients with sleep-disordered breathing and CHF. A recent study demonstrated that at 1-year follow-up there is a statistically significant higher recurrence rate of atrial fibrillation after cardioversion in patients with untreated SAHS compared with treated SAHS (82% vs. 42%).

27. What is the role of cardiac pacing in SAHS?

The role of atrial pacing in SAHS remains unclear. A recent study of 15 patients who required permanent atrial-synchronous ventricular pacemakers for symptomatic bradycardia demonstrated that atrial overdrive pacing (15 beats above the mean nocturnal sinus rate) decreased the AHI from a mean of 28 to a mean of 11. There was improvement in both central and obstructive apneas. The AHI returned to baseline values when the pacemaker was turned off. The exact mechanism by which atrial overdrive pacing improves sleep-disordered breathing remains to be elucidated. Whether cardiac pacing improves apneas and hypopneas in patients without indications for pacemaker or significant cardiac disease remains to be determined.

SAHS AND ISCHEMIC HEART DISEASE

28. Does SAHS increase the risk of ischemic heart disease?

The Sleep Heart Health Study reported a weak but statistically significant association between sleep-disordered breathing and self-reported ischemic heart disease with an odds ratio of 1.27.

ST-segment changes due to myocardial ischemia are fairly common in patients with coronary artery disease and SAHS. Myocardial ischemia is related to the severity of both SAHS and coronary artery disease. Nocturnal myocardial ischemia may lead to nocturnal angina or silent ischemia. No clear evidence indicates that SAHS causes nocturnal myocardial ischemia without concomitant coronary artery disease. SAHS in patients with coronary artery disease has been associated with a worse long-term prognosis. CPAP has been shown to improve nocturnal angina and ischemic ST-segment changes in uncontrolled studies. Randomized, controlled trials are necessary to evaluate the role of CPAP in patients with ischemic heart disease and SAHS.

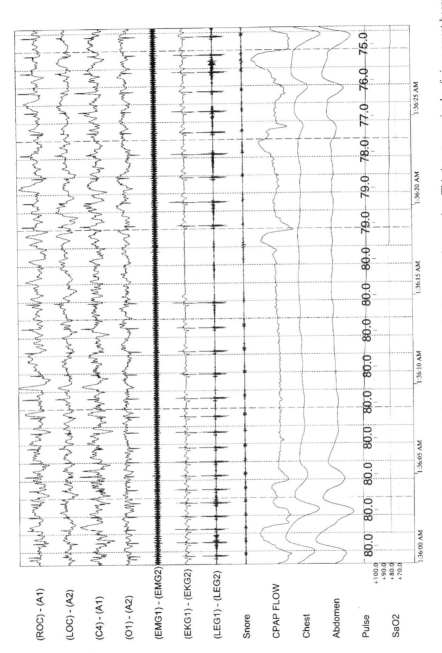

Figure 2. An episode of severe sinus bradycardia with pause during an apneic event with oxygen desaturation. This is not an episode of sinus arrest because the eventual QRS complex is not a junctional escape beat and is preceded by a normal P wave. This episode actually occurred during CPAP titration.

SAHS AND STROKE

29. Does SAHS increase the risk of ischemic stroke?

The Sleep Heart Health Study, a large population-based, cross-sectional study, demonstrated a modest association between SAHS and stroke. The odds ratio of stroke was 1.58 times higher in patients with AHI $\geq$ 11 than in patients with AHI $\leq$ 1.4, suggestive of a dose relationship between the severity of SAHS and stroke.

30. How common is SAHS after stroke?

SAHS, defined as AHI $\geq$ 10, occurs in 69% to 90% of patients who have suffered a stroke. In fact, many stroke victims have moderate-to-severe SAHS. One prospective study demonstrated no significant difference in the AHI acutely after stroke and at 3 months of follow-up. Therefore, SAHS most likely precedes the cerebrovascular accident. Central sleep apnea, although reported, is much less common than SAHS in this group of patients.

31. Does SAHS affect the outcome of patients who have suffered an ischemic cerebrovascular accident?

Yes. SAHS has an independent adverse outcome on the recovery of patients with stroke. Several studies have reported that the presence of SAHS (AHI $\geq$ 10) in stroke patients was associated with worse functional impairment and a longer period of hospitalization and rehabilitation compared with patients with similar extent of stroke without SAHS.

BIBLIOGRAPHY

1. Bassetti C, Aldrich MS: Sleep apnea in acute cerebrovascular diseases: Final report on 128 patients. Sleep 22:217–223, 1999.
2. Becker HF, Jerrentrup A, Ploch T, et al: Effect of nasal continuous positive airway pressure treatment on blood pressure in patients with obstructive sleep apnea. Circulation 107:68–73, 2003.
3. Bradley TD, Floras JS: Sleep apnea and heart failure. Part I: Obstructive sleep apnea. Circulation 107:1671–1678, 2003.
4. Bradley TD, Floras JS: Sleep apnea and heart failure. Part II: Central sleep apnea. Circulation 107:1822–1826, 2003.
5. Garrigue S, Bordier P, Jais P, et al: Benefit of atrial pacing in sleep apnea syndrome. N Engl J Med 346:404–412, 2002.
6. Kanagala R, Murali NS, Friedman PA, et al: Obstructive sleep apnea and the recurrence of atrial Fibrillation. Circulation 107:2589–2594, 2003.
7. Kaneko Y, Floras JS, Usui K, et al: Cardiovascular effects of continuous positive airway pressure in patients with heart failure and obstructive sleep apnea. N Engl J Med 348:1233–1241, 2003.
8. Kaneko Y, Hajek VE, Zivanovic V, et al: Relationship of sleep apnea to functional capacity and length of hospitalization following stroke. Sleep 26:293–297, 2003.
9. Leung RS, Bradley TD: Sleep apnea and cardiovascular disease. Am J Respir Crit Care Med 164:2147–2165, 2001.
10. Nieto FJ, Young TB, Lind BK, et al: Association of sleep-disordered breathing, sleep apnea, and hypertension in a large community-based study. Sleep Heart Health Study. JAMA 283:1829–1836, 2000.
11. Peppard PE, Young T, Palta M, et al: Prospective study of the association between sleep-disordered breathing and hypertension. N Engl J Med 342:1378–1384, 2000.
12. Shahar E, Whitney CW, Redline S, et al: Sleep-disordered breathing and cardiovascular disease: Cross-sectional results of the Sleep Heart Health Study. Am J Respir Crit Care Med 163:19–25, 2001.

18. SLEEP AND MEDICAL DISORDERS

Jim Cygan, MD

1. What is the most common sleep complaint in patients with asthma and chronic obstructive pulmonary disease?

Patients with asthma and chronic obstructive pulmonary disease (COPD) frequently complain of difficulty in sleep initiation and maintenance, poor sleep quality, and excessive daytime sleepiness. The above symptoms may or may not be related to airway obstruction or medication effect.

2. What factors predict nocturnal hypoxemia in patients with COPD?

Several factors contribute to hypoxemia. Changes in chemoresponsiveness to carbon dioxide result in decreased ventilation for a given physiologic increase in carbon dioxide during sleep. The end result is a decrease in minute ventilation secondary to a decrease in tidal volume with subsequent hypoxemia. Due to decreased accessory muscle tone, especially during rapid-eye-movement (REM) sleep, there is a decline in functional residual capacity (FRC), which causes a worsening ventilation/perfusion ratio that results in nocturnal desaturations. Some authors have found the following parameters to be possible predictive indexes of nocturnal desaturations: high body mass index (BMI), reduced forced expiratory volume in one second (FEV_1), or elevated diurnal partial pressure of carbon dioxide (pCO_2). Concurrent sleep apnea-hypopnea syndrome (SAHS) in patients with COPD is a factor that contributes to nocturnal hypoxemia. The incidence may be as high as 15%.

3. Is thyroid function testing indicated in all patients with SAHS?

The answer to this question is highly controversial. (See questions 4 and 5).

4. Summarize the arguments in favor of thyroid function testing in all patients with SAHS.

Physiologic mechanisms have been proposed to explain possible causes of sleep apnea in patients with hypothyroidism, including reduced upper airway patency due to myxedematous infiltration of tissue, impaired function of upper airway muscles, and reduced central drive to upper airway muscles. The diagnosis of hypothyroidism and treatment with thyroid replacement therapy may preclude the need for polysomnography (PSG) and/or possible titration of continuous positive airway pressure (CPAP). Thyroid replacement, with or without CPAP therapy, eventually reverses the underlying cause of the patient's obstructive sleep apnea.

5. Summarize the arguments against thyroid function testing in all patients with SAHS.

Routine testing may result in false-positive results, leading to possible further testing and/or inappropriate treatment. Such problems can increase the cost-benefit ratio compared with not performing routine testing. In addition, several studies have shown that in the absence of (1) signs or symptoms of hypothyroidism, (2) persistent symptoms with adequate CPAP therapy, or (3) disproportionately more severe symptoms than expected for severity of sleep-disordered breathing, thyroid screening does not appear to be necessary. The prevalence of hypothyroidism appears to be similar in patients with suspected or confirmed SAHS and in the general population.

6. Does SAHS cause diabetes mellitus?

The possibility of an association is still debated, but if present, the association appears to be weak. Data indicate that hypertensive, obese men with severe SAHS have an increased risk of diabetes mellitus, although obesity appears to be the main risk factor. After correction for confounding factors, however, there still appears to be a slight increase in risk. In addition, limited data have shown that plasma insulin levels can be elevated in sleep-disordered breathing and that these elevated levels may or may not be associated with obesity.

7. What disorder of growth hormone regulation is associated with SAHS?

Acromegaly. The prevalence of SAHS in acromegaly, as documented in several small studies, ranges from 39% to 91%. The pathophysiology of sleep apnea in this disease has not clearly been identified, but several mechanisms have been suggested. Macroglossia is probably not an important etiologic factor, but craniofacial changes associated with acromegaly may play a role. Central respiratory depression may contribute as a cause of the central apneas that have been documented with this disorder.

8. What role does menopause play in sleep disorders?

The data related to the effect of vasomotor responses (i.e., hot flashes) associated with menopause and their impact on sleep are mixed. Less efficient sleep, secondary to increased arousals by hot flashes, has been documented in menopausal women, and treatment with estrogen replacement therapy may decrease these sleep disturbances. Other studies, however, have shown that sleep quality is not improved with estrogen replacement therapy in menopausal women with hot flashes. Although not clearly elucidated, causes of insomnia other than hot flashes include mood disorders and sleep-disordered breathing. A recent large cohort study has found menopause to be an independent risk factor for SAHS.

9. What is the relationship of gastroesophageal reflux disease and SAHS?

The data related to the frequency of gastroesophageal disease (GERD) in patients with SAHS is mixed. Some studies document that patients with SAHS have a high frequency of GERD, with rates ranging from 50% to 70%, whereas others find no association between SAHS and GERD. One possible mechanism of nocturnal reflux is increased gastric pressures during periods of upper airway obstruction and a subsequent increase in breathing effort and abdominal pressure. Of interest, treatment with continuous positive airway pressure has been shown to improve nocturnal GERD in patients with SAHS.

10. What sleep disorders are seen in patients with inflammatory bowel disease?

Data related to patients with inflammatory bowel diseases and sleep disorders are scarce. The only two published studies concluded the following: (1) patients with inflammatory bowel disease dream about their bowels and about soiling themselves significantly more often than a control population, and (2) patients with ulcerative colitis treated with intravenous cyclosporine vs. total colectomy have improved sleep quality.

11. What sleep disorders are seen in patients with irritable bowel syndrome?

Patients with irritable bowel syndrome have a subjectively significant increase in nonrestful sleep and insomnia associated with increased daytime fatigue. But objective data from PSG studies do not show differences in sleep architecture compared with controls. Apparently, the poor sleep is associated with daytime psychological stress. In addition, poor sleep may also be associated with worsening of diurnal gastrointestinal symptoms in this patient population.

12. What sleep complaints are seen in patients with rheumatoid arthritis?

Complaints such as unrefreshing sleep and daytime somnolence, resulting from insomnia and/or sleep apnea, have been noted in patients with rheumatoid arthritis. Both central and obstructive sleep apneas have been reported in patients with rheumatoid arthritis. Vertical subluxation of the odontoid process can compress the brainstem and result in central sleep apnea. Changes in the temporomandibular joint and/or position of the cervical vertebrae can occur in rheumatoid patients and may give rise to narrowing of the upper airway, resulting in obstructive sleep apnea. Although pain is the presumed cause of initiation and maintenance insomnia in this patient population, the converse may also be true; that is, sleep disruption may worsen the diurnal pain syndrome experienced in patients with rheumatoid arthritis.

13. What sleep complaints are commonly seen in patients with fibromyalgia?

Patients with fibromyalgia report early morning awakenings, awakening feeling tired or unrefreshed, and initiation and/or maintenance insomnia. Case reports have documented an increased frequency of SAHS in patients with fibromyalgia compared with the general population. However, larger, prospective, controlled trials are needed to confirm this association.

14. Do patients in the intensive care unit have normal sleeping pattern?

No. Sleep disturbances commonly occur in patients during an intensive care unit (ICU) admission. Both subjective surveys and PSG measurements in patients in the ICU reveal numerous causes of disturbed sleep as well as sleep architecture abnormalities. Patient sleep is disrupted due to increased noise (staff talking, telemetry alarms), vital sign measurements, phlebotomy, medication effects, lighting, and frequent interventions by medical personnel. PSGs from ICU patients reveal poor sleep efficiency, increased wake time, increased NREM stage 1 sleep, increased awakenings, and decreased slow-wave sleep and REM sleep.

15. Does the mode of mechanical ventilation affect a patient's sleep in the ICU?

According to one study, pressure support ventilation is more disruptive to patients than assist-control ventilation. Although the patients receiving either type of mechanical ventilation had fragmented sleep, the patients receiving pressure support ventilation had more awakenings during sleep. The primary cause of the awakening was secondary to central apneas. Arousals and awakening can be associated with catecholamine and blood pressure changes, which may be detrimental to patients in the ICU. In addition, ambulatory patients with a similar degree of sleep disturbance have decreases in attention, short-term memory, and verbal recall. Such deficits, if occurring in intubated ICU patients, may prolong the weaning process.

16. Are sleep disturbances common in pregnancy?

Sleep disturbances are reported in more than 70% of pregnant women and include daytime sleepiness and insomnia. In general, women experience increasing daytime sleepiness, insomnia, nocturnal awakenings, and worse sleep quality as the pregnancy progresses. During the second trimester, however, the majority of women report normalization of sleep pattern.

17. What causes the sleep disturbances in pregnancy?

The causes are myriad and result from both hormonal and secondary medical/physical changes that occur during pregnancy. The interaction of estrogen and progesterone during pregnancy, although not fully elucidated, can cause both insomnia and daytime sleepiness. For instance, estrogen is known to decrease REM sleep. Other hormones that probably play a role in sleep disturbances in pregnant women include cortisol, melatonin, and prolactin. Insomnia, especially during the third trimester, has been reported secondary to fetal movement, abdominal discomfort, leg cramps, GERD, nocturia, and backache.

18. Do pregnant patients commonly develop SAHS with weight gain during pregnancy?

Although case reports document the development of SAHS during pregnancy, large, controlled, prospective studies are not available to verify this association. In a small trial comparing PSGs of obese pregnant women with nonobese pregnant women, results showed a statistically significant increase in the apnea-hypopnea index (AHI) in both populations at 12 week sand 30 weeks of gestation. However, the mean AHIs in the obese and nonobese pregnant patients were within the normal range (AHI < 5) at both time points.

19. Are pregnant women at risk for nocturnal hypoxemia?

Small studies have demonstrated nocturnal desaturations in healthy pregnant patients with uncomplicated pregnancies, independent of obstructive sleep apnea, but the clinical significance is unknown. Diurnal measurements of pulmonary function in pregnant women reveal a reduction in FRC secondary to an elevated diaphragm from the enlarged uterus. In sleep, a physiologic decrease in FRC may be further compounded by the pulmonary mechanics described above and may result in a decrease in maternal oxygenation. Concomitantly, protective physiologic changes in pregnancy, such as increased minute ventilation from elevated circulating progesterone and a right shift of the oxyhemoglobin desaturation curve, may protect the mother and fetus from nocturnal desaturations.

20. Do sleep disturbances occur in cirrhotic patients?

Small studies have reported several sleep disturbances in patients with subclinical hepatic encephalopathy, including delayed sleep onset, delayed wake-up time, increased nocturnal awakening, and a propensity for increased nocturnal activities. These disturbances appear to correlate with disease onset in comparison to a cirrhotic-free population. The etiology of these sleep abnormalities is speculative, but small human and animal studies have demonstrated disruption of the diurnal rhythm of melatonin as a possible cause of sleep disturbances in cirrhotic patients.

21. What sleep disorder is most commonly associated with end-stage renal disease?

SAHS, periodic limb movement disorder (PLMD), restless leg syndrome (RLS), and insomnia have been reported frequently in patients on dialysis. The prevalence of these disorders exceeds 50% in the majority of studies. Both obstructive and central sleep apneas occur in patients with chronic renal failure and often do not develop until the onset of renal failure. The etiology of apnea in this population is speculative, but several possible causes include nocturnal breathing dysregulation due to chronic metabolic acidosis and an elevated blood urea nitrogen (BUN) level, upper airway edema due to the fluid overload state often seen in patients with renal disease, and reduced perioropharyngeal muscle tone due to uremia. The source of PLMD/RLS is probably metabolically induced from the pH, electrolyte, and BUN abnormalities. The etiology of insomnia in end-stage renal disease is most likely multifactorial and possibly includes PLMD/RLS, sleep apnea, and metabolic disturbances.

22. How can SAHS be treated in patients with chronic renal failure on dialysis?

Hemodialysis, without continuous positive airway pressure (CPAP) therapy, may improve SAHS. Two small, prospective, randomized studies comparing conventional diurnal hemodialysis (3 days/week) with daily nocturnal hemodialysis demonstrated a statistically significant decrease in the AHI in the nocturnal hemodialysis group. In neither of the studies did the AHI reach the normal range, and in one of the studies the change in BUN directly correlated with improvement in AHI. Of note, there was no correlation between a decreasing BUN level and a decrease in PLMD. Mechanisms that may explain the improvement in sleep apnea with nocturnal dialysis were not explored in these studies. The most reasonable explanation may be the decrease in extracellular volume associated with more frequent dialysis.

23. Do sleep disturbances occur in blind patients?

In a large prospective, control-matched study, using a comprehensive questionnaire to determine the impact of blindness on the sleep/wake pattern, revealed increased nocturnal sleep disruption and daytime somnolence in patients with visual loss. The degree of visual disturbance (i.e., blindness) did not correlate with the severity of sleep disturbance. Bright light is believed to be the strongest environmental factor that influences the biologic clock. Since light/photic information, via the retinohypothalamic tract, is conveyed from the retina to the circadian pacemaker in the suprachiasmatic nucleus, it was speculated that visual loss may disturb this pathway and contribute to a "free-running pacemaker" and/or simply disturbed sleep. In another smaller, prospective, controlled study, the authors used pineal gland production of melatonin as a surrogate for the integrity of retinohypothalamic pathway since melatonin secretion is determined by retinal input of light (at night plasma concentrations are higher compared with the day). In 3 of 11 blind patients, bright light suppressed plasma melatonin levels—a normal response. Consequently, the physiologic mechanisms that contribute to disturbed sleep/wake cycle in blind patients are complex and not fully understood.

24. How commonly do patients with cancer have sleep disturbances? What are the most common disturbances?

Most studies related to sleep in cancer patients are small, lack objective data, and focus on a sole cancer. One study, however, included a large cross-sectional survey that used sleep questionnaires to identify the prevalence of sleep disturbances in patients with a large variety of cancers. The mean prevalence rates in all patients for leg restlessness, insomnia, and excessive sleepiness were 41%, 31%, and 28%, respectively. Most patients had chronic insomnia (> 6 months), with onset shortly after the cancer diagnosis. Factors associated with insomnia were mood changes, restless legs, and use of sleeping pills. Another smaller study, using objective data, described the sleep characteristics in patients with lung and breast cancer. The most significant finding in this study was the prevalence of periodic limb movement disorder in 47% of patients with lung cancer and 60% of patients with breast cancer. Other factors, in general, that may contribute to disturbed sleep in patients with cancer include cancer therapy (chemotherapy and radiation treatment), depression, pain, anxiety, and metabolic/endocrine changes associated with cancer and its treatment.

BIBLIOGRAPHY

1. Davidson JR, MacLean AW, Brundage MD, Schulze K: Sleep disturbance in cancer patients. Soc Sci Med 54:1309–1321, 2002.
2. Gabor JY, Cooper AB, Hanly PJ: Sleep disruption in the intensive care unit. Curr Opin Crit Care 7:21–27, 2001.
3. Grunstein RR: Acromegaly and sleep apnea. Ann Intern Med 115:527–532, 1991.
4. Hanly PJ, Pierratos A: Improvement of sleep apnea in patients with chronic renal failure who undergo nocturnal hemodialysis. N Engl J Med 344:102–107, 2001.
5. Ing AJ, Ngu MC, Breslin ABX: Obstructive sleep apnea and gastroesophageal reflux. Am J Med 108:120S–125S, 2000.
6. McNicholas WT: Impact of sleep in COPD. Chest 117:48S–53S, 2000.
7. Martin RJ, Banks-Schlegel S: Chronobiology of asthma. Am J Respir Crit Care Med 158:1002–1007, 1998.
8. Santiago JR, Nolledo MS, Kinzler W, Santiago TV: Sleep and sleep disorders in pregnancy. Ann Intern Med 134:396–408, 2001.
9. Tabandeh H, Lockley SW, Buttery R, et al: Disturbance of sleep in blindness. Am J Ophthalmol 126:707–712, 1998.
10. Winkelman JW, Goldman H, Piscatelli N, et al: Are thyroid function tests necessary in patients with suspected sleep apnea? Sleep 19:790–793, 1996.
11. Young T, Finn L, Austin D, Peterson A: Menopausal status and sleep-disordered breathing in the Wisconsin Sleep Cohort Study. Am J Respir Crit Care Med 167:1181–1185, 2003.

19. SLEEP AND NEUROLOGIC DISORDERS

Suzanne Stevens, MD

EPILEPSY

1. What is the effect of sleep deprivation on epileptiform activity?

Sleep deprivation has been associated with lowering the seizure threshold and increasing epileptiform activity on the electroencephalogram (EEG). It is used as a provocation for seizures on epilepsy monitoring units and is employed before clinical EEGs in an attempt to bring out epileptiform abnormalities. Sleep deprivation may be a component of worsening seizure control when sleep fragmentation is due to SAHS, periodic limb movement disorder, or other primary sleep disorder. However, one recent study in an inpatient population with severe seizure disorders found that sleep deprivation was not provocative.

2. What stage of sleep is thought to be protective against epileptiform activity?

Rapid-eye-movement (REM) sleep is thought to be protective against epileptiform activity due to its mixed frequency and lack of synchronization.

3. What stage of sleep is thought to promote epileptiform activity?

Slow-wave sleep is thought to promote epileptiform activity due to its high-frequency, synchronizing waveforms.

4. Define simple partial seizures.

Simple partial seizures involve a limited region of the cortex. The manifestation can be motor impairment (i.e., jacksonian seizure) or sensory impairment. The seizure may manifest as an emotional or hallucinatory (visual, auditory, olfactory) phenomenon, epigastric rising, déjà vu, or jamais vu. Consciousness is maintained during a simple partial seizure as opposed to impairment of consciousness during a complex partial seizure.

5. Define complex partial seizures.

Complex partial seizures involve an alteration of consciousness due to bilateral spread of the seizure discharge. Complex partial seizures often are accompanied by automatisms, such as lip smacking or other perseverative movements. A typical complex partial seizure out of sleep is shown in Figure 1.

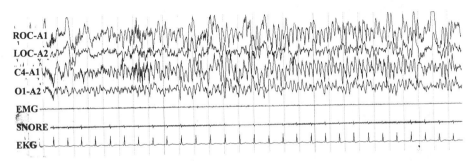

Figure 1. A typical PSG recording showing evolving, rhythmic epileptiform activity in the ocular, central, and occipital leads. The EEG changes are more prominent in the right-sided leads, and repetitive movements were noted in the left hand. The motor activity is not shown on this recording.

6. Define generalized seizure.

A generalized seizure involves tonic-clonic activity of the extremities.

7. Is an EEG abnormality necessary for the diagnosis of a seizure?

No. A seizure is a clinical diagnosis.

8. What percentage of patients have only nocturnal seizures?

Ten percent of seizure patients are thought to have only nocturnal seizures without daytime seizures.

9. What types of seizure disorders occur most often at night?

Benign focal epilepsy of childhood with rolandic spikes, juvenile myoclonic epilepsy, electrical status epilepticus during sleep (continuous spikes and waves during sleep), and some frontal lobe seizures, such as nocturnal paroxysmal dystonia and autosomal dominant frontal lobe seizures.

10. At what time of day do the abnormalities of juvenile myoclonic epilepsy become more apparent both clinically and on the EEG?

Juvenile myoclonic epilepsy (JME), or myoclonic epilepsy of Janz, may have large myoclonic jerks that tend to occur in the morning after awakening. In addition, generalized seizure may occur, again more commonly in the morning hours.

11. Describe the typical EEG abnormalities of juvenile myoclonic epilepsy.

EEG shows polyspike and spike-and-wave discharges that are synchronized and symmetric. They tend to be seen in the transitions into sleep and while awakening. However, the abnormalities are not seen during sleep.

12. What is autosomal dominant nocturnal frontal lobe epilepsy?

Autosomal dominant nocturnal frontal lobe epilepsy (ADNFLE) is an inherited form of frontal lobe epilepsy with a focus on chromosome 8.

13. Does EEG monitoring always reveal abnormal findings during a frontal lobe seizure?

No. Frontal lobe seizures often have normal EEG findings. In addition, clinical manifestations of frontal lobe seizure may be atypical, such as nonstereotypic vocalizations and asynchronous extremity movements. The index of suspicion must be high, and frontal lobe seizures must be included in the differential diagnosis of all patients presenting with atypical seizure.

14. Define nocturnal paroxysmal dystonia.

Nocturnal paroxysmal dystonia (NPD) occurs during non-REM sleep and is a dystonic or choreoathetoiod movement of the extremities. NPD is now thought to represent a frontal lobe seizure, which can occur exclusively during sleep.

15. How is nocturnal paroxysmal dystonia diagnosed?

Often NPD is a clinical diagnosis because EEG and polysomnography (PSG) are usually normal.

16. What is the typical age of onset of nocturnal paroxysmal dystonia?

Onset may occur at any time from infancy to the fifth decade of life.

17. Describe the natural history of nocturnal paroxysmal dystonia.

Untreated patients can have NPD for years without progression. Treated patients typically respond well to pharmacotherapy.

18. What treatment options are available for nocturnal paroxysmal dystonia?

Patients typically respond well to antiepileptic medications, particularly carbamazepine.

19. Describe the typical EEG findings of nocturnal paroxysmal dystonia.
Typically the EEG is normal.

MOVEMENT DISORDERS

20. What movement disorders may persist during sleep?
- Secondary palatal myoclonus is known to persist during sleep.
- The tremor of Parkinson disease (PD) has been recorded during stage I sleep but is not present in other stages of sleep.
- Tics have been seen during sleep.

21. What is head-banging?
Head-banging, or jactatio capitis nocturna, is more common in children than adults and occurs during the transition from sleep to wake. It is a rhythmic forward-backward movement that can persist even into light non-REM sleep. Head-banging is classified under rhythmic movement disorder (see below).

22. When do rhythmic movement disorders occur?
Rhythmic movement disorder occurs during the transition from sleep to wakefulness and from wakefulness to sleep.

23. What happens to the tremor of Parkinson disease during sleep?
The resting tremor of PD typically improves with consolidated sleep but can return when the patient is aroused to lighter stages of non-REM sleep.

24. Do the tics of Tourette syndrome persist during sleep?
Yes. The tics can persist during all stages of sleep but generally decrease in frequency once pharmacotherapy is started.

25. How is head-banging treated?
Treatment with clonazepam may improve the condition.

26. How does sleep affect primary palatal myoclonus?
Primary palatal myoclonus often improves during sleep, whereas secondary palatal myoclonus (due to an underlying lesion) often persists during sleep.

27. How is rhythmic movement disorder treated?
Patients may benefit from treatment with benzodiazepines for muscle-relaxant effects and sleep initiation and consolidation.

NEUROMUSCULAR DISEASES

28. What major neuromuscular disorders may cause sleep disturbances?
Amyotrophic lateral sclerosis (ALS), myasthenia gravis, and several forms of muscular dystrophy may be associated with sleep disorders. Multiple sclerosis, although not a neuromuscular disorder, also may be associated with sleep effects. In addition, diaphragmatic paralysis, due to several different causes, can cause sleep complaints.

29. What type of sleep disorder is most commonly reported in patients with neuromuscular disorders?
Several different sleep disorders may be present in this population. Both central apneas, possibly due to central nervous system effects of the underlying disease, and obstructive apneas/hypopneas may be present. The obstructive apneas appear to be due to the muscle weakness of both upper airway and respiratory muscles caused by the underlying disease.

30. What is the most common complaint in patients with neuromuscular disorders?

Patients may complain of symptoms similar to those of other patients with sleep apnea-hypopnea syndrome (SAHS). Morning headache may be especially prominent. Acute orthopnea—shortness of breath within seconds of assuming the supine position—is especially suggestive of diaphragm dysfunction.

31. Can the presence of sleep disorders in patients with neuromuscular disorders be predicted?

In general, the more severe the underlying disease, the more likely that a sleep disorder is present, but there is great variability among patients. Patients with a neuromuscular disorder and coexistent lung disease are especially at risk.

32. What historical and physical examination findings suggest an underlying sleep disorder?

Daytime ventilatory dysfunction predisposes patients to nocturnal breathing disorders. Insomnia, hypersomnia, or other features of disturbed sleep may be a strong indicator of sleep-disordered breathing.

33. How do the sleep effects of myotonic dystrophy differ from the sleep effects of other neuromuscular diseases?

Patients with myotonic dystrophy appear to have a greater severity of daytime sleepiness than patients with other neuromuscular diseases. The reason remains unknown.

34. What testing is indicated for evaluating a patient with neuromuscular disease and possible sleep-disordered breathing?

Overnight polysomnography is indicated to exclude nocturnal breathing events in patients suspected of sleep-disordered breathing. In addition, abnormalities of daytime pulmonary function testing and arterial blood gases may indicate a risk for nocturnal hypoventilation.

35. What is the best treatment for patients with neuromuscular disease?

Supplemental oxygen may improve oxygen desaturation, although patients' symptoms may not improve. In addition, continuous positive airway pressure (CPAP) improves sleep-disordered breathing. If obstructive events are treated with CPAP and oxygen saturations remain low, bilevel positive airway pressure (BiPAP) may enhance ventilation.

DEMENTIA

36. What is the most common sleep complaint of patients with dementia?

Patients with dementia generally complain of circadian rhythm disruption, which causes wakefulness during the night and sleeping during the day. This problem is generally of greater concern when dementia is in the more severe stages, because it may increase caregiver burden.

37. How are circadian sleep complaints treated?

Treatment of circadian sleep problems associated with dementia includes increasing light exposure during daytime hours, restricting daytime napping, and increasing daytime social interactions and physical activity to promote improved nighttime sleep.

38. Define sundowning.

Sundowning is defined as the nighttime confusion and agitation that may occur with dementia. It often affects the caregiver significantly; sundowning is a common reason for institutionalizing patients with dementia.

39. How is sundowning treated?

Antipsychotic medictations such as haloperidol, clozapine, olanzapine, and respiridone are used for the treatment of sundowning in dementia. Melatonin is a promising alternative, although further studies are needed.

40. What effect does dementia have on the EEG?

Dementia can cause slowing of the background activity to include more theta activity, making staging of sleep more difficult. In addition, decreased spindle activity has been noted.

41. What changes in sleep architecture are commonly seen with dementia?

Common changes in sleep architecture include higher percentage of stage I sleep, lower sleep efficiency, and increasing awakenings, all of which indicate poor quality of sleep. These abnormalities seem to worsen with more severe dementia.

42. Describe the relationship between sleep apnea-hypopnea syndrome and dementia.

The prevalence of SAHS and clinically significant SAHS is unknown in this population. However, if SAHS is suspected clinically on the basis of symptoms, PSG should be performed. SAHS may be more common in vascular dementia than in other categories of dementia.

43. What obstacles are encountered in the treatment of SAHS in patients with dementia?

Patients with dementia may not tolerate CPAP well—particularly if they are prone to sundowning, which worsens nighttime confusion. If patients have difficulty with using CPAP, a supportive caregiver or family member who can help them during the nighttime hours may improve compliance.

44. What types of dementia are associated with REM sleep behavior disorder?

Patients with diffuse Lewy body disease, which is associated with dementia, parkinsonism, and hallucinations, are more prone to develop REM sleep behavior disorder (RBD). This population is at particularly high risk for injury that can result from RBD. RBD is much less common in Alzheimer's disease.

STROKE

45. How can a stroke affect sleep?

Patients may present with a variety of sleep complaints following stroke. Hypersomnia can occur after damage to specific areas of the brain (see below). Insomnia may be a common complaint, usually not related to the localization of the stroke. Vivid dreaming and/or hallucinations have been reported following vascular lesions, particularly in the pedunculi (peduncular hallucinosis), pontomesenchephalic tegmentum, mesencephalic tegmentum, and paramedian thalamus.

46. How are snoring, sleep apnea, and stroke associated?

Snoring has been considered a risk factor for stroke. Although studies have shown a high prevalence of SAHS in the early and chronic stroke populations, at this point research has not found strong supporting evidence that treatment of SAHS influences long-term outcome in rehabilitation. Studies investigating the relationship between SAHS and stroke must control for obesity and hypertension, which are risk factors for both stroke and SAHS.

47. Does SAHS precede stroke, and does stroke cause SAHS?

SAHS can either precede stroke or be caused by stroke. Brainstem lesions resulting from the vascular injury of stroke are particularly susceptible to causing SAHS if the nerves supplying the pharyngeal musculature are involved.

48. Does location of the stroke increase the risk of having SAHS?

In the studies done to date, location does not predict the finding of SAHS in patients with stroke. However, there have been case reports of SAHS following bulbar stroke. Central apnea was not a prominent feature in such patients; the events were obstructive.

49. Does stroke severity predict the presence of SAHS?

In the studies done to date, severity of stroke does not predict the presence of SAHS following stroke.

50. What sleep disorders have been reported after a stroke?
Numerous sleep-related complaints have been reported after stroke, including insomnia, hypersomnia, periodic limb movement disorder, SAHS, and RBD. RBD is typically reported following vascular lesions of the brainstem. When a patient presents with insomnia following stroke, depression must be considered in the differential diagnosis.

51. What disorders have been reported with thalamic strokes?
There have been reports of hypersomnia in strokes affecting the bilateral paramedian thalamus.

52. What EEG change may result from a stroke in the thalamus?
Ipsilateral loss of spindles has been reported with thalamic lesions after stroke.

53. At what time of day are patients most likely to have a stroke?
Patients are more likely to have a stroke between the hours of 6 AM and noon, similar to the pattern seen with myocardial infarction.

54. How prevalent is obstructive sleep apnea among stroke patients?
In the largest study to date, Bassetti et al. found SAHS in 62.5% of stroke patients compared with 12.5% of the control group. SAHS was defined as an apnea-hypopnea index (AHI) > 10.

55. Discuss theories about the relationship between obstructive sleep apnea and stroke.
Enhanced platelet aggregation during the night and generally increased aggregability in the morning hours may contribute to the development of thrombosis. Fibrinogen levels in stroke patients with SAHS are increased. In addition, SAHS causing increased intracranial pressure coupled with decreased systemic blood pressure leads to decreased cerebral perfusion pressure, possibly compromising blood flow.

PARKINSONIAN DISORDERS

56. How prevalent are complaints about sleep among patients with Parkinson disease?
Up to 90% of patients with Parkinson disease (PD) have complaints of sleep disturbance.

57. What changes in sleep architecture have been reported in patients with Parkinson disease?
Patients with PD have shown reduced total sleep time, reduced sleep efficiency, and increased wakenings as well as increased arousals compared with a control population. Inconsistent findings have included reduced slow-wave sleep and reduced REM sleep.

58. What are the typical sleep complaints in patients with Parkinson disease?
Patients with PD may complain of insomnia, hypersomnia, awakenings due to stiffness with difficulty in changing positions, and nocturia.

59. How do dopaminergic medications influence sleep?
Dopaminergic medications have been implicated as a cause of daytime sleepiness after the initial report of a patient with PD who had a motor vehicle accident while on a dopamine agonist. Similar reports followed. No large-scale, placebo-controlled clinical trials have confirmed this finding in larger numbers of patients.

60. What side effects associated with sleep may be seen in patients who take dopaminergic medications?
- Dopaminergic agents can cause vivid dreams as well as hallucinations. In fact, hallucinations may represent abnormal REM phenomena.
- In some patients dopaminergic agents have been reported to cause insomnia, which may resolve upon changing to another agent in the same class of medications.

- Additional parasomnia behavior such as sleep-talking and sleep-walking have been reported with dopaminergic medications.

61. Describe the relationship between REM sleep behavior disorder and Parkinson disease.

RBD is found in at least 15% of patients with PD. It can be a cause of injury. RBD is characterized by patients' acting out their dreams. Dream content generally becomes more vivid and involves themes of chasing people or being attacked. Patients with RBD are more likely to have hallucinations, indicating that REM abnormalities are common to both RBD and hallucinations.

62. Describe the relationship between restless legs syndrome and Parkinson disease.

The prevalence of restless legs syndrome (RLS) in patients with PD is unknown, but it is common in this population. RLS can be associated with difficulty in initiating and maintaining sleep.

63. Describe the relationship between periodic limb movement disorder and Parkinson disease.

Both periodic limb movement disorder (PLMD) and PD are thought to be due to dopaminergic abnormalities in the central nervous system, and both can be treated with dopaminergic medications. PLMD is found frequently in patients with PD; the prevalence is thought to be around 30%.

64. How common is SAHS in patients with Parkinson disease?

The prevalence is unknown.

65. How common is excessive daytime sleepiness in patients with Parkinson disease?

Excessive daytime sleepiness (EDS) has been reported in up to 15–50% of patients with PD. Although causes may be multifactorial, dopaminergic medication has been implicated as causing daytime sleepiness, resulting in motor vehicle accidents and decreased quality of life. Other possible causes of EDS in patients with PD include central nervous system dysfunction and fragmented nighttime sleep. In addition, given its high incidence in patients with PD, depressison should be considered as well.

66. What are the effects of subthalamic nuclei stimulation?

In one study, patients showed increased sleep efficiency and longer total sleep time after implantation of a subthalamic nucleus stimulator.

67. What behavioral treatments are used in patients with Parkinson disease and sleep disorders?

Sleep hygiene measures include regular exercise and avoidance of caffeine late in the day. If nocturia is a contributing factor, limiting fluid intake in the hours prior to bedtime may improve the problem. Naps should be avoided, particularly late in the day, to avoid interfering with nocturnal sleep initiation.

68. What pharmacologic measures may improve sleep disorders in patients with Parkinson disease?

Nocturnal bradykinesia or rigidity may benefit from nocturnal doses of dopaminergic medication, unless the medication causes insomnia. In patients with nocturnal hallucinations and confusion, atypical neuroleptic medication may be helpful. If RBD is present, treatment with clonazepam or shorter-acting benzodiazepine may be helpful. To date, melatonin has not been proved to be of benefit, but large-scale trials are lacking.

PRION DISEASES

69. What is a prion?

A prion is a protein that invades cells and replicates by using the cell's DNA. The prion itself has no DNA or RNA for replication.

70. List examples of prion diseases that affect the central nervous system.
- Creutzfeldt-Jakob disease (CJD)
- Gerstman-Sträussler-Scheinker (GSS) syndrome
- Kuru
- Fatal familial insomnia (FFI)

71. What is Creutzfeldt-Jakob disease?
Named after two German psychiatrists, Hans Gerhard Creutzfeldt and Alfons Maria Jakob, CJD is a rare disease associated with various mutations of the prion protein gene. It occurs in sporadic (85–95%), familial, and infectious forms.

72. What are the signs and symptoms of Creutzfeldt-Jakob disease?
Signs include varying degrees of spongiform degeneration of neurons, neuronal loss, gliosis, and amyloid plaque formation. These findings are accompanied by rapidly progressive dementia, myoclonus, motor disturbances, and characteristic changes in the EEG. Death usually occurs within 1 year of onset, although courses up to 5 years are not uncommon.

73. What is Gerstmann-Sträussler-Scheinker syndrome?
GSS syndrome is a group of rare prion diseases of autosomal dominant inheritance. They have the common characteristics of cognitive and motor disturbances with multicentric amyloid plaques in the brain. Death occurs within 1–3 years of onset.

74. What is kuru?
Kuru, which means "shivering" in the language of the Fore people of New Guinea, is an infectious prion disease with a long incubation period. It is found only among the Fore and neighboring peoples of New Guinea and is believed to be associated with ritualistic cannibalism. Symptoms include truncal and limb ataxia, a shivering-like tremor, and dysarthria. Kuru inevitably ends in death.

75. Describe the presentation of fatal familial insomnia.
This rare disease presents with severe, progressive insomnia, eventually culminating in total lack of sleep. Additional symptoms include cognitive changes with stuporous episodes and autonomic manifestations such as hyperhidrosis, tachycardia, tachypnea, hypertension, hypersalivation, urinary problems, constipation, and impotence. Further symptoms seen as the disease progresses include dysarthria, hyperreflexia, ataxia, and myoclonus.

76. What is the course of fatal familial insomnia?
The course progresses rapidly. Death occurs within 7–32 months from onset of symptoms.

77. How is fatal familial insomnia transmitted genetically?
FFI is transmitted in an autosomal dominant manner.

78. What is seen pathologically in the brains of patients with fatal familial insomnia?
The anterior and dorsomedial thalamic nuclei show severe atrophy and neuronal loss with reactive gliosis. Other thalamic nuclei are far less affected.

79. What does polysomnography show in patients with fatal familial insomnia?
PSG initially may show slowing of, followed by loss of, normal background activity. As the disease progresses, virtually no slow-wave sleep is detected, and near the end stages of the disease, only a few minutes of sleep can be recorded during 24 hours. In addition, EEG has shown periodic sharp waves in the end stages of the disease.

HEADACHE

80. What is the significance of morning headache?

Morning headaches have many potential causes. They are not specific for one particular sleep disorder. Causes include sinusitis, brain tumor, migraine, chronic obstructive pulmonary disease, and tension headaches. Morning headaches also may be associated with obstructive sleep apneas, insomnia, or hypersomnia.

81. How common are morning headaches in SAHS?

Approximately 20-50% of patients with SAHS complain of morning headache. The mechanism may be due to hypercapnia or sleep fragmentation.

82. What is a hypnic headache?

Hypnic headache is a very rare type of headache occurring solely during sleep. It has been documented to occur usually out of REM sleep. Patients describe it as excruciatingly painful, similar to cluster headaches without the autonomic symptoms.

83. How is hypnic headache treated?

Patients may benefit from prophylactic treatment with verapamil or lithium.

84. What is the association between cluster headaches and SAHS?

If SAHS associated with cluster headaches is treated with CPAP, the cluster headaches improve significantly.

85. How does sleep affect migraine?

Sleep deprivation is a known provocative factor for migraines. In addition, during a migraine headache attack, sleep is known to improve the symptoms of the migraine.

BIBLIOGRAPHY

1. Bourke SC, Gibson GJ: Sleep and breathing in neuromuscular disease. Eur Respir J 19:1194–1201, 2002.
2. Chokroverty S: Sleep, breathing and neurologic disorders. In Chokroverty S (ed): Sleep Disorders Medicine, 2nd ed. Boston, Butterworth-Heinemann, 1999, pp 509–565.
3. Comella CL: Sleep disturbances in Parkinson's disease. Curr Neurol Neurosci Rep 3:173–180, 2003.
4. Deuschl G, Wilms H: Palatal tremor: The clinical spectrum and physiology of a rhythmic movement disorder. Adv Neurol 89:115–130, 2002.
5. Kohyama J, Matsukura F, Kimura K, Tachibana N: Rhythmic movement disorder: Polysomnographic study and summary of reported cases. Brain Devel 24:33–38, 2002.
6. Krachman SL, Criner GJ: Restrictive lung diseases and neuromuscular disease. In Lee-Chiong TL, Sateia MJ, Carskadon MA (eds): Sleep Medicine, Philadelphia, Hanley & Belfus, 2002, pp 329–338.
7. Mendez M, Radtke RA: Introductions between sleep and epilepsy. J Clin Neurophysiol 18:106–127, 2001.
8. Mohsenin V: Sleep-related breathing disorders and risk of stroke. Stroke 32:1271–1278, 2001.

20. SLEEP PHARMACOLOGY

James J. Herdegen, MD

DISORDERS OF INITIATING AND MAINTAINING SLEEP

1. What symptoms occur with benzodiazepine withdrawal syndrome?

The benzodiazepine withdrawal syndrome encompasses a number of clinical symptoms:
- **Central nervous system:** rebound insomnia, irritability, panic attacks, difficulty with concentrating, anxiety, psychotic reactions, seizures
- **Gastrointestinal:** dry retching, nausea
- **Cardiovascular:** palpitations
- **Systemic:** muscle pain and stiffness, diaphoresis, weight loss, hand tremor

2. Which sedative-hypnotic drug is most commonly prescribed for insomnia?

Historically, sedative-hypnotic drugs known as benzodiazepines have been the major class of drugs used to treat insomnia, the most popular of these being triazolam (Halcion). Although the clinical efficacy of current benzodiazepines such as triazolam has been well established, these agents are associated with unwanted side effects such as memory impairment and next-day residual sedation. In the late 1980s, a new class of drugs was developed, known as the nonbenzodiazepines. They have a reduced side-effect profile compared with the benzodiazepines. Zolpidem (Ambien), a member of the nonbenzodiazepine class, is the market leader in the United States with more than $900 million in sales in 2001. A number of other medications currently under development are expected to improve on side-effect profiles or to be better tolerated in target populations such as the elderly.

3. How should benzodiazepine dosing be adjusted for patients with chronic lung disease?

Short half-life sedative hypnotic medications (zaleplon, zolpidem) taken at their recommended doses have been shown to be reasonably safe in patients with chronic obstructive pulmonary disease (COPD). A randomized, placebo-controlled trial found no significant change in mean oxygen saturation or greater percent time less than 90%. Long-acting drugs (e.g., flurazepam, flunitrazepam) may cause a significant decrease in arterial partial pressure of oxygen (PaO_2) and an increase in arterial partial pressure of carbon dioxide ($PaCO_2$). Therefore, when sedative-hypnotic medication is considered, drugs with a shorter half-life are preferred.

4. How should benzodiazepine dosing be adjusted for patients with chronic liver disease?

Some benzodiazepine medications undergo enzymatic inactivation by microsomal oxidation through the liver. Factors that influence the degradation of medications through the microsomal enzyme system include age, liver disease, and the concomitant use of other medications (such as cimetidine, erythromycin, estrogens, and some of the selective serotonin reuptake inhibitors). A different subset of benzodiazepines (lorazepam and temazepam) is inactivated by hepatic glucuronide conjugation, which is not affected by age, liver disease, and competing drug effects. Therefore medication type, coexisting liver disease, and drug half-life are important factors to consider in prescribing benzodiazepine medications. In patients with chronic liver disease, a good general rule is to use short half-life medications that are not dependent on microsomal enzyme degradation.

5. How should benzodiazepine dosing be adjusted for elderly patients?

The elderly population represents about 35% to 40% of prescriptions for sedative-hypnotic agents. Benzodiazepine receptor agonists may increase the risk of falling in the elderly and often have a significantly prolonged half-life. When such medications are initiated in the elderly, the lowest possible dose should be considered, along with use of agents with a shorter half-life. For example, the initial dose of temazepam should be 7.5 mg.

6. What are the long-term effects of sedative-hypnotic use in patients with insomnia?

Nightly use of benzodiazepines is recommended for no longer than 4 weeks. This recommendation is made because chronic administration may lead to **physiologic and possibly psychological dependence**. Physiologic dependence is associated with withdrawal syndrome on discontinuation. Shorter-acting drugs produce an earlier and more intense withdrawal syndrome compared with longer-acting drugs and in general produce more withdrawal problems. Withdrawal syndrome can last as little as 1-4 days, as long as 2 weeks, or can lead to a longer-term persistent phenomenon. Because withdrawal symptoms are often the same as presenting symptoms, it is difficult to determine whether they are a side effect of drug use or merely a return of insomnia symptoms.

Drug tolerance, a reduction in pharmacologic effects with repeated administration, is another possible consequence of long-term use. Tolerance is linked to the changes in receptor binding that occur with chronic administration. Compared with the older sedative hypnotics, such as the barbiturates, tolerance to the hypnotic effects of benzodiazepines is minimal if they are used for less than 4 weeks. No evidence of tolerance has been observed with zolpidem or zaleplon (selective benzodiazepine receptor agonists), even with use as long as 179 and 365 days, respectively.

7. How do benzodiazepines affect sleep architecture?

Benzodiazepine receptor agonists, depending on their onset of action, usually shorten sleep latency, reduce arousals or nocturnal awakenings, and increase total sleep time. The nonselective benzodiazepine agonists alter normal sleep patterns by prolonging light sleep and reducing both slow-wave sleep and REM sleep. Rebound insomnia (prolonged sleep onset and waking after sleep onset) may occur after drug withdrawal. Benzodiazepines also have a significant effect on the microarchitecture of the sleep electroencephalogram (EEG) by suppressing activity in the low-frequency range and increasing activity in the spindle-frequency range.

8. How does the onset of action differ among sedative-hypnotic agents?

There can be significant variability in the onset of action and half-life of medications despite the drug class commonality, as shown in the table below.

Characteristics of Sedative-Hypnotic Medications

Agent	Trade Name	Dosage (mg)	Onset of Action (min)	Half-life (hr)
Zaleplon	Sonata	5–20	30	1
Zolpidem	Ambien	5–10	30	1.5–4.5
Trazodone	Desyrel	50–150	30–60	5–9
Temazepam	Restoril	15–30	45–60	3–25
Clonazepam	Klonopin	0.5–2	20–60	19–60

9. Do sedative-hypnotic drugs increase the risk of motor vehicle accidents?

A number of studies have documented deficits in cognition and attentiveness as well as physiologic sleepiness, as measured by the multiple sleep latency test (MSLT), especially after using long-acting benzodiazepines. One study of outpatients in Great Britain found that patients taking benzodiazepines were more likely to have automobile accidents when medicated. This finding was not observed for patients taking antidepressants or phenothiazines. Another study found that 5% of Finnish drivers involved in automobile accidents had significant blood concentrations of diazepam compared with 2% of controls. However, these population studies were unable to control for potential confounding factors, such as an inherently greater risk of traffic accidents in patients who receive sedative-hypnotic agents, regardless of the medication itself.

10. What is the role of melatonin in the treatment of insomnia?

Melatonin, athough not approved by the Food and Drug Administration (FDA), is a hormone available over the counter as a sleeping aid. When used in doses of 0.1–0.5 mg, it produces blood levels in the physiologic range. When given at the right time of day, it appears to have a role in shifting circadian rhythms and inducing sleepiness. For example, to shift the endogenous circadian rhythm to an earlier time (phase advance), melatonin is ingested in the late afternoon to early evening. Taking melatonin in the morning produces a shift of rhythms to a later time. This phase-shifting effect provides the rationale for the use of melatonin to treat jet lag syndrome, delayed sleep phase syndrome, and the non–24-hour sleep-wake disorder of blind people.

The use of melatonin for insomnia, despite evidence of sleepiness and sleep-promoting effects, is less well established. Some but not all controlled studies have demonstrated clinical efficacy. There continues to be no consensus on the recommended dosage, time of administration, indications, and contraindications.

11. How do the newer hypnotic agents, zaleplon and zolpidem, differ from older agents?

The nonselective benzodiazepines act as classic agonist compounds at the gamma-aminobutyric acid (GABA)- benzodiazepine receptor complex, binding to benzodiazepine receptors (BZ1 and BZ2). Benzodiazepines also have muscle-relaxant, anxiolytic, and anticonvulsant properties. These properties may be related to their binding to BZ2 and BZ3 receptor subtypes.

DISORDERS OF EXCESSIVE DAYTIME SLEEPINESS

12. What was the first stimulant used for narcolepsy?

Amphetamine use was first proposed in 1935, but amphetamines have fallen out of favor due to drug tolerance, side effects, high addictive potential, and potential risk in pregnancy.

13. What stimulants are useful for the treatment of narcolepsy?

The stimulants used for narcolepsy include amphetamines, methylphenidate, and pemoline. Characteristics of these different medications are shown in the table below. These medications cause central nervous system stimulation of major midbrain dopamine systems, leading to enhanced release and reuptake blockade of norepinephrine, dopamine, and serotonin.

Characteristics of Stimulant Medications

Agent	Receptor Type	Half-life (hr)	Time to Maximum Level (hr)	FDA Indication	Scheduling
Modafinil	Unknown	15	2-4	Yes	IV
Amphetamines	Dopamine agonist	10 SR: 15+	2 SR: 8–10	Yes/selected agents	II
Methylphenidate	Dopamine agonist	4 SR: 8–10	2 SR: 5	Yes/selected agents	II
Pemoline	Dopamine agonist	12	2–4	No	II

SR = sustained release.

14. How is sodium oxybate useful in the treatment of narcolepsy?

Sodium oxybate is the first medication approved by the FDA for the treatment of cataplexy associated with narcolepsy. It significantly reduces cataplexy attacks and improves excessive daytime sleepiness (EDS) as reported using the Epworth sleepiness scale. The effect on EDS may be a result of improved sleep consolidation and slow-wave sleep.

15. What medications are useful in treating cataplexy in patients with narcolepsy?

Medications for cataplexy include the tricyclic antidepressants (TCAs), serotonin reuptake inhibitors (SSRIs), venlafaxine, and sodium oxybate. The antidepressants are postulated to act through inhibition of rapid-eye-movement (REM) phenomena, and the anticataplectic effect correlates with inhibition of norepinephrine reuptake.

16. How does modafinil differ from traditional stimulant medications?

Modafinil is chemically unrelated to central nervous system stimulants. It causes activation of hypothalamic regions but does not act directly through dopaminergic pathways. It may indirectly inhibit GABA release.

17. Which stimulant medications lead to a positive result on urine drug screens?

A urine drug screen is typically positive in patients taking amphetamines. The result is often positive if sampling occurs within 24 to 48 hours of drug ingestion.

18. What monitoring is essential for patients treated with pemoline?

In rare cases, pemoline can cause severe hepatotoxicity, at times fatal. For this reason the manufacturer recommends liver function monitoring every 2 weeks.

RESTLESS LEGS SYNDROME/ PERIODIC LIMB MOVEMENT SYNDROME

19. What drugs are approved by the FDA for the treatment of restless legs syndrome (RLS) or periodic limb movement syndrome (PLMS)?

No medications are currently approved by the FDA for the specific treatment of RLS or PLMS. Thus all medications are used "off label," despite a number of clinical studies looking at treatment outcomes.

20. Which antidepressants have been shown to worsen RLS?

The tricyclic antidepressants and serotonin reuptake inhibitors have been associated with worsening RLS symptoms.

21. Which antidepressants have been shown to worsen PLMS?

Antidepressant medications have been clinically reported to exacerbate RLS or associated PLMS, thereby worsening sleep problems. Paradoxically, some patients report benefit from these medications. Although no studies have clearly addressed these issues, the treating physician should be aware of the potential of tricyclic antidepressants and serotonin reuptake inhibitors (SSRIs), such as fluoxetine (Prozac) and sertraline (Zoloft), to aggravate RLS and PLMS. If the history suggests that prescription medications may be exacerbating RLS symptoms, appropriate alternatives should be recommended; however, it may be necessary to coordinate with the patient's health care providers to ensure comprehensive, effective treatment of any comorbid conditions.

22. Which dopaminergic agent appears to be the best for treatment of PLMS?

Dopamine agonists (DAs) bind to dopamine receptors, producing dopamine-like effects. These medications include the ergot derivatives bromocriptine mesylate (Parlodel) and pergolide mesylate (Permax) and the nonergotoline drugs pramipexole dihydrochloride (Mirapex) and ropinerole hydrochloride (Requip). As with several treatment regimens used to treat RLS, most DAs were developed as anti-parkinsonian agents. Levodopa treatment alone was found to cause side effects, including rebound and augmentation. DAs are much less likely to cause these side effects and are currently preferred over the use of levodopa.

The DAs are currently recommended for patients with RLS who have mild-to-severe symptoms sufficient to impair quality of life. DAs may be used as first-line therapies in patients with moderate or severe RLS or as appropriate alternatives or supplements to carbidopa/levodopa. The preferred dopaminergic agent for PLMS remains controversial given the paucity of comparative studies. If a patient is found to demonstrate clinical response to dopaminergic agents with few side effects, the use of pramipexole may be an appropriate first-line drug based on its half-life and side-effect profile.

23. By what mechanism can metoclopromide and prochlorperazine worsen RLS?

Both agents are dopamine antagonists and appear to mediate an increase in RLS symptoms through this mechanism. Although the increase is thought to be caused by central dopamine antagonistic properties because of their sedating properties, there may be some effect on peripheral receptors also.

PREGNANCY

24. Discuss the safety profile of different stimulants in pregnancy.

The use of stimulants during pregnancy should be avoided if possible since little safety information is available. Amphetamine abuse may increase the incidence of cardiac defects and cleft palate and lead to infant withdrawal symptoms. Pemoline is the only category B medication; all others are in category C.

Category B indicates that animal studies do not indicate a risk to the fetus and that no controlled human studies are available or that animal studies show an adverse effect on the fetus but that well-controlled studies in pregnant women have failed to demonstrate a risk to the fetus. Category C indicates that studies have shown that the drug exerts animal teratogenic or embryocidal effects, although no controlled studies are available in women, or that no studies are available in either animals or women.

25. Discuss the safety profile of different agents used for RLS/PLMD in pregnancy.

None of the drugs used to treat RLS are known to be safe in pregnancy; in many cases, no information at all is available. Nonpharmacologic measures, therefore, are the safest treatments for women who experience RLS during pregnancy. In addition, if such patients are experiencing symptomatic RLS associated with iron deficiency, iron supplementation may be particularly helpful. Because RLS typically becomes more severe as the pregnancy progresses, drug therapy may often be withheld until the third trimester, at which time such medications have the least risk of causing teratogenic effects. Carbamazepine, especially, is contraindicated in the first semester. In regard to specific medications, pergolide is a category B medication; all others are in category C.

DRUGS OF ABUSE

26. What are the long-term effects of alcohol on sleep architecture?

Studies in alcoholics who have become abstinent show that the effects of alcohol on sleep architecture—decreased amounts of slow wave sleep and REM sleep—can persist from several months to many years after abstinence. Even in nonalcoholics, moderate drinking 6 hours before bedtime can affect sleep architecture by lowering the amounts of stage I and REM sleep. A number of studies have investigated the effect of alcohol administration to alcoholic patients undergoing inpatient treatment for alcoholism. In most of these studies, alcohol resulted in difficulty in falling asleep (prolonged sleep latency), decreased total sleep time, increased percentage of slow-wave sleep, decreased percentage of REM sleep, and increased REM sleep latency.

In studies of alcoholics during withdrawal, sleep latency remained increased and total sleep time remained decreased compared with baseline levels. However, slow-wave sleep percentage and REM sleep latency decreased during withdrawal relative to drinking nights and returned to baseline levels. REM sleep percentage increased during withdrawal

27. What are the effects of acute alcohol ingestion on polysomnogram results?

Alcohol is a central nervous system depressant that leads to a sympathetic arousal state after the decline in blood alcohol levels. Acute alcohol administration enhances adenosine activity which in turn inhibits the acetylcholine system. Because acetylcholine contributes to REM sleep, alcohol-induced increases in adenosine activity may play a role in decreasing REM sleep following alcoholic intoxication. During alcohol withdrawal, adenosine activity is lower than normal, which favors arousal and excessive REM sleep (known as REM rebound).

28. Is alcohol effective for the treatment of insomnia?

Several studies have estimated that 6-19% of the general population and 15–28% of people with insomnia have used alcohol to promote sleep. Alcohol has sedative properties that can reduce the sleep latency onset. However, alcohol is not a reliably effective sedative among alcoholic patients; the improved sleep quality in drinking patients is confined primarily to the first week of drinking. This finding appears to be due to a rapid tolerance effect, along with frequent fragmentation of sleep after the alcohol is cleared.

29. What are the long-term effects of cocaine use on sleep architecture?

In small clinical studies of cocaine users, the acute use of cocaine caused a suppression of REM sleep; during drug withdrawal a rebound of REM is seen that is not seen in other stages of sleep. REM variables subsided to normal levels on the third recovery night following cocaine use.

Another study described the sleep of nine patients admitted to an inpatient substance abuse treatment unit. The patients' sleep was studied in the laboratory for 4 nights during the first week and 2 nights during the second and third weeks of hospitalization. During the first week of withdrawal, patients had a markedly shortened REM latency, an increased REM sleep percentage, a very high REM density, and a long total sleep period time. During the third week, REM latencies were very short and total percentage of REM sleep was increased. By week three of withdrawal, the sleep continuity pattern was similar to that found in chronic insomnia, with a long sleep latency, an abnormally increased total time awake after sleep onset, and poor sleep efficiency.

30. What are the effects of cocaine on MSLT results?

If patients are undergoing abrupt withdrawal at the time of the overnight sleep study and MSLT, a significantly reduced sleep latency and REM latency would be expected. Many laboratories routinely obtain urine drug screening at the time of the MSLT for this reason.

31. Does opiate abuse lead to central sleep apnea?

Several studies have described an increased incidence of central sleep apnea in patients undergoing treatment with opiates for chronic pain syndromes and patients receiving methadone as part of a drug treatment program. It is likely that illegal opiate use will produce similar effects.

MISCELLANEOUS ISSUES

32. What is meant by the term *Prozac eyes*?

Fluoxetine (Prozac) and other selective serotonin reuptake inhibitors have been associated with significantly more eye movements and arousals during non-REM sleep compared with control groups. In one study, these saccadic eye movements in non-REM sleep were detected in 48.8% of patients taking fluoxetine.

33. Do other agents cause this phenomenon?

The effect of fluoxetine on non-REM eye movements is postulated to derive from potentiation of inhibitory serotonergic neurons, leading to disinhibited saccadic eye movements. Therefore, any medication that potentiates serotonin release or prevents reuptake may also lead to saccadic eye movements. Other medications may include phenothiazines, antiepileptic medications such as phenytoin (Dilantin), and benzodiazepines.

34. What medications commonly increase EEG spindle activity?

Benzodiazepine receptor agonists, especially if taken on a chronic basis, often lead to increased spindle activity. Halothane, which decreases pontine acetycholine release, has been described to increase EEG spindle activity, along with barbiturates.

35. How does steroid therapy affect sleep architecture?

Use of corticosteroids, such as prednisone, has been associated with psychologic disturbances, including euphoria, insomnia, personality changes, severe depression, and frank psychosis. The primary effect on sleep is increased wake time after sleep onset. In a study of healthy volunteers receiving 4 days of prednisone, polysomnography revealed an increase in central theta-wave brain electrical activity, which returned to baseline following prednisone withdrawal. This effect was directly correlated with prednisone-induced increases in subjective sadness ratings and with decreases in self-rated energy and well-being. Prednisone-induced reductions in peak alpha-wave activity were also directly correlated with increases in subjective sadness and Symptom Checklist-90 ratings and with decreases in self-rated hypomanic symptoms.

Androgenic steroids have been associated with an increase in sleep apnea in men. Hormone replacement therapy in perimenopausal women may reduce hot sweats and therefore reduce arousals and wake time after sleep onset.

BIBLIOGRAPHY

1. Aleksy LM, Smith MA: Sedatives and hypnotics in lactation. J Human Lactat 14:61–64, 1998.
2. Borgen LA, et al: Sodium oxybate (GHB) for treatment of cataplexy. Pharmacotherapy 22:798–799, 2002.
3. Hening W, et al: The treatment of restless legs syndrome and periodic limb movement disorder: An American Academy of Sleep Medicine Review. Sleep 22:970–999, 1999.
4. Holbrook AM, et al: Meta-analysis of benzodiazepine use in the treatment of insomnia. Can Med Assoc J 162:225–233, 2000.
5. Hoover-Stevens S, Kovacevic-Ristanovic R: Management of narcolepsy in pregnancy. Clin Neuropharmacol 23(4):175–181, 2000.
6. Lenhart SE, Buysse DJ: Treatment of insomnia in hospitalized patients. Ann Pharmacother 35:1449–1457, 2001.
7. Lippman S, Mazour I, Shahab H: Insomnia: Therapeutic approach. South Med Assoc J 94:866–873, 2001.
8. Littner M, et al: Practice parameters for the treatment of narcolepsy: An update for 2000. Sleep 24:451–466, 2001.
9. Mitler MM, Hayduk R: Benefits and risks of pharmacotherapy for narcolepsy. Drug Safety 25:791–809, 2002.
10. Murray L, Seger D: Drug therapy during pregnancy and lactation. Emerg Med Clin North Am 12:129–149, 1994.
11. Obermeyer WH, Benca RM: Effects of drugs on sleep. Neurol Clin 14:827–840, 1996.
12. Parrino L, Terzano MG: Polysomnographic effects of hypnotic drugs: A review. Psychopharmacologia 126:1–16, 1996.
13. Weimerskirch PR, Ernst ME: Newer dopamine agonists in the treatment of restless legs syndrome. Ann Pharmacother 35:627–630, 2001.
14. Wincor MZ: Melatonin and sleep: A balanced view. J Am Pharmaceut Assoc 38:228–229, 1998.
15. Wortelboer U, et al: Tolerability of hypnosedatives in older patients. Drugs Aging 19:529–539, 2002.

IV. Pediatric Sleep

21. PEDIATRIC POLYSOMNOGRAPHY

Jean Silvestri, MD, and Debra Weese-Mayer, MD

INDICATIONS

1. Which pediatric sleep disorders require polysomnography to make a diagnosis?

Polysomnography (PSG) is recommended to differentiate benign primary snoring from sleep apnea/hypopnea syndrome (SAHS), to determine the nature and severity of alveolar hypoventilation syndromes, and to evaluate children with disturbed sleep patterns, excessive daytime sleepiness, cor pulmonale, or failure to thrive.

The PSG is also used to make the diagnosis of SAHS in children with other confounding disorders such as sickle cell disease, cystic fibrosis, bronchopulmonary dysplasia, or neuromuscular disease. Although polysomnography is not necessary to make a diagnosis, PSG is useful in children with laryngomalacia whose symptoms are worse during sleep and children who have cor pulmonale or failure to thrive. PSG is also used to titrate the adequacy of artificial ventilation whether by tracheostomy or noninvasive ventilation with mask continuous positive airway pressure (CPAP) or bilevel ventilation.

2. When should patients with suspected rapid-eye-movement (REM) and non-REM parasomnias be evaluated with polysomnography?

Several manifestations of non-REM partial arousal disorders are common in childhood. Children may simply sit up during sleep or quietly sleep walk, but they may also have confusional arousals or even sleep terrors. Typically the diagnosis is made from the clinical description. Polysomnography is nonspecific unless the child has a characteristic spell during the study.

Polysomnography is indicated in some cases when injury to the child may occur, when the spells may result from other sleep-related disorders, when it is necessary to differentiate non-REM parasomnias from sleep-related seizure activity, or when medication is being considered. REM parasomnias, nightmares, and REM-sleep motor disorder can be distinguished from non-REM disorders on the basis of clinical data. However, polysomnography can be considered when behavioral intervention does not resolve the symptoms, medication is being considered, or an accurate diagnosis is needed.

3. Describe the role of home polysomnography in pediatric patients.

Overnight polysomnography in a pediatric respiratory physiology laboratory is the gold standard for diagnosis. However, resources may be limited, and the need for unattended sleep studies and home recordings is increasing. Unfortunately, limited data are available for validation of home recordings, whether they include oximetry only or multichannel recordings, especially in the unattended setting of the home.

4. Which pediatric patients undergoing tonsillectomy and adenoidectomy should be evaluated with polysomnography?

In order to determine which patients require surgery and to determine the severity of physiologic compromise, a PSG is recommended. The PSG can be used to determine whether intensive postoperative monitoring is indicated.

ELECTROENCEPHALOGRAPHY

5. At what age does slow-wave sleep typically develop?

Slow-wave sleep becomes predominant during the first part of the night at about three months of age.

6. How are sleep states divided for infants?

According to the newborn infant sleep manual by Anders, Emde, and Parmelee, sleep is divided into active-REM sleep, quiet sleep, and indeterminate sleep. Active-REM sleep occurs when the eyes are closed, but there is a large amount of activity including smiles, grimaces, sucking, or even limb movements. Rapid eye movements are noted, electromyographic (EMG) activity is low and respiration is irregular. During quiet sleep, body movements are not noted, respirations are regular, EMG activity is low, and rapid eye movements are not recorded. Indeterminate sleep does not meet criteria for either of the other two categories.

7. How does sleep architecture typically differ in pediatric patients compared with adults?

Sleep architecture is different in pediatric patients and adults but also changes over the first years of life. A full-term infant has sleep onset in active sleep and short sleep cycles. The percentage of active sleep is high: 60% in the full-term infant. This percentage decreases to approximately 30% by 6 months of age. This decrease is associated with a concomitant increase in quiet sleep from about 49% at 3 months to about 55% at 6 months. By 2 years of age, non-REM sleep occurs after sleep onset, REM sleep decreases to adult levels, and non-REM/REM sleep cycle duration increases to adult values of about 90 minutes.

8. Rechtschaffen and Kales scoring criteria are used beginning at what age?

The criteria of Rechtschaffen and Kales are typically used to stage sleep in infants 6 months of age and older. Under 6 months, the distinction between quiet and active sleep is usually adequate.

RESPIRATORY MEASUREMENTS

9. How is expired carbon dioxide measured in pediatric polysomnography?

Expired carbon dioxide is measured by end-tidal carbon dioxide monitoring with a catheter placed at the nose or mouth. Care must be taken to ensure that the catheter remains patent and that there is a good waveform with a plateau. If a patient has an increased respiratory rate or obstructive lung disease, the waveform may be unreliable. If there are difficulties with this measurement, transcutaneous carbon dioxide monitoring can be used. The transcutaneous modality does not reflect acute changes but can provide trends over time.

10. Why is expired carbon dioxide used in pediatric polysomnography?

Oxygenation and ventilation are vital indicators of physiologic compromise; hence it is essential that hemoglobin saturation and end-tidal carbon dioxide be measured continuously during pediatric polysomnography. Coupled with inductance plethysmography of the chest and abdomen, these channels allow detection of hypoventilation as well as apnea. Recognizing that pediatric patients most typically have partial upper airway obstruction rather than complete airway obstruction, these channels are essential to the diagnosis of the condition and to the determination of the severity of physiologic compromise. Observation of the child's ventilatory and arousal responses to endogenous challenges of hypoxemia and hypercarbia are also important in characterizing the extent of physiologic compromise.

ARTIFACTS

11. What causes recording artifacts in pediatric patients?

Recording artifacts are unavoidable. Artifacts may be related to the patient, the equipment, or the environment. For this reason a skilled technician must closely monitor the study.

12. Which artifacts are most common in pediatric patients?
- The most common artifact is the 60-hertz interference, which can result from any electrical equipment.
- Electrocardiography (EKG) artifact is common and may be due to the strong electrical field from cardiac activity and proximity to the field of recording electrodes.
- Pulse artifact is also seen as an artifact in phase with the cardiac cycle on the flow channel.
- Movement artifact is quite common and typically is viewed across all channels.
- Sucking artifact, usually seen in infants and young children, is recorded as the waxing and waning of the chin EMG tone.
- There may be intentional or patient-generated artifacts.

All of these artifacts demonstrate the need for close observation and meticulous documentation throughout the recording.

BIBLIOGRAPHY

1. American Thoracic Society: Standards and indications for cardiorespiratory sleep studies in children. Am J Respir Crit Care Med 153:866–878, 1996.
2. Crowell DH , for the CHIME Study Group: An Atlas of Infant Polysomnography. New York, Parthenon Publishing Group, 2003.
3. Curzi-Dascalova L, Challamel M-J: Neurophysiological basis of sleep development. In Loughlin GM, Carroll JL, Marcus CL (eds): Sleep and Breathing in Children: A Developmental Approach. New York, Marcel Dekker, 2000, pp 3–37.
4. Rosen GM, Mahowald MW: Disorders of arousal. In Loughlin GM, Carroll JL, Marcus CL (eds): Sleep and Breathing in Children: A Developmental Approach. New York, Marcel Dekker, 2000, pp 333–345.
5. Sheldon SH, Riter S, Detrojan M: Atlas of Sleep Medicine in Infants and Children. Armonk, NY, Futura Publishing Company, 1999.

22. PEDIATRIC INSOMNIA: LIMIT-SETTING SLEEP DISORDER AND SLEEP-ONSET ASSOCIATION DISORDER

Lisa J. Meltzer, PhD, and Jodi A. Mindell, PhD

LIMIT-SETTING SLEEP DISORDER

1. What is limit-setting sleep disorder?

Limit-setting sleep disorder occurs when parents or caretakers inconsistently enforce bedtime limits, resulting in bedtime stalling or refusing to go to bed at an appropriate time. These inconsistencies at bedtime result in delayed sleep onset and decreased overall sleep time.

2. How common is limit-setting sleep disorder?

Bedtime resistance is found in 10–30% of toddlers and preschoolers. However, limit-setting sleep issues can also be found in older children. According to parents' reports in one study, 15% of children aged 4–10 years have problematic bedtime resistance.

3. What is the difference between bedtime refusal and bedtime stalling?

In **bedtime refusal** a child refuses to get ready for bed, go to bed, or stay in bed after lights are out. In **bedtime stalling** a child attempts to delay bedtime by requesting additional activity time (e.g., watching television, reading books) or seeking attention from parents after bedtime (e.g., curtain calls). Children quickly learn which requests will elicit a positive response from parents (e.g., requests for the potty, one more hug), and these requests become frequent bedtime-stalling techniques.

4. What are the symptoms of limit-setting sleep disorder?

Children with limit-setting sleep disorder either refuse to go to bed or attempt to delay the bedtime. Once asleep, their sleep quality and quantity are normal. Specific symptoms include (1) ignoring or refusing to comply with parental requests to get ready for bed, (2) refusing to go to bed or requiring a parent to sit with the child while he or she falls asleep, (3) frequent requests for parental attention after bedtime (e.g., "curtain calls," requests for hugs, drinks), and (4) delaying child's sleep onset 30 minutes or more.

5. Is limit-setting sleep disorder associated with the child's age?

Yes. Toddlers and preschoolers are learning to assert their independence, which can result in increased noncompliance at bedtime. As children grow older, parental involvement at bedtime typically decreases, thus decreasing the opportunity for problematic limit setting.

6. Does limit-setting sleep disorder only occur at bedtime?

No. It can also occur during the day (at naptime).

7. How do parents contribute to limit-setting sleep disorder?

Parents can contribute to limit-setting sleep disorder in three ways. First, limit-setting problems occur when parents place few, if any, limits on the child's sleep behaviors (e.g., the child watches television in the bedroom while falling asleep). Second, parents may set limits in an unpredictable or inconsistent manner, which reinforces and maintains the child's behavior. Finally, parental responses to inappropriate behaviors (e.g., allowing a child a third trip to the bathroom within 10 minutes) can contribute to limit-setting sleep disorder.

8. How can one determine whether parental limit-setting is contributing to the child's sleep problems?

When the child is able to go to bed and fall asleep quickly for others (e.g., babysitter, grandparent) or falls asleep quickly at the desired bedtime in other situations (e.g., falls asleep watching television in living room at designated bedtime), this suggests that parental limit-setting contributes to the child's sleep problems.

9. What environmental factors contribute to limit-setting sleep disorder?

Limits can be difficult to set when the child shares a bedroom with his or her parents or siblings. In addition, parents of children with current or past medical problems may have difficulty in setting limits due to feelings of guilt or concerns that the child is vulnerable.

10. Is one parenting style more common in limit-setting sleep disorder?

A permissive parenting style, in which parents generally set few, if any, limits on their child's behavior, can result in limit-setting sleep disorder.

11. If parents have conflicting discipline styles, how does this conflict affect bedtime behaviors?

When parents disagree about how to handle behavioral issues, children can sense that one parent is more strict while the other is more lenient. This situation can result in increased noncompliant behaviors because the child may exploit this conflict between parents.

12. Do children with limit-setting sleep disorder also have frequent night wakings?

Yes. Night wakings are common in children with limit-setting sleep disorder, a result of either limit-setting issues during the night or negative sleep associations (e.g., parental presence) at bedtime, as described below.

13. Discuss the relationship between limit-setting sleep disorder and daytime behavior problems.

In general, children who are "poor sleepers" have increased daytime behavior problems. This finding may be a result of inadequate sleep and/or the possibility that parents who have difficulty in setting limits on negative behaviors at bedtime may also have inconsistent limit-setting during the day.

14. When should a child be referred for treatment of limit-setting sleep disorder?

When bedtime problems are persistent, severe, or disruptive of the family, the child (or adolescent) should be referred to a mental health or sleep professional who can address the behavioral issues contributing to the child's sleep problems.

15. If left untreated, what are the consequences of limit-setting sleep disorder?

Bedtime struggles, if untreated, can result in daytime behavior problems (as discussed above), family tension, and bedtime problems that are persistent and unchanging.

16. Are behavioral management techniques effective?

Yes. Effective behavioral techniques include establishing appropriate sleep habits (e.g., set bedtime, consistent bedtime routine) and appropriate limit setting (e.g., clear bedtime rules, ignoring complaints/protests, being persistent and consistent).

17. What different behavioral management techniques should be suggested to parents for limit-setting sleep disorder?

Behavior management techniques can include (1) using positive reinforcement (e.g., praise) to increase desired behaviors, (2) avoiding punishment to decrease negative behaviors, (3) being consistent in responding, (4) giving commands instead of questions ("Time for bed" vs. "Are you ready for bed?"), (5) setting clear limits and following through, and (6) providing acceptable choices that are within reasonable limits ("Do you want to go to bed now or in 5 minutes?").

18. Are medications indicated in the treatment of limit-setting sleep disorder?

No. Given that limit-setting sleep disorder is due to either inconsistent parenting or environmental factors, medications are not indicated for treatment.

19. What is the prognosis for children with limit-setting sleep disorder?

With appropriate behavioral interventions, limit-setting sleep disorder can be typically well-controlled. In addition, parents who learn appropriate limit-setting skills at bedtime often generalize these skills to daytime behaviors as well.

SLEEP-ONSET ASSOCIATION DISORDER

20. What is sleep-onset association disorder?

Sleep-onset association disorder occurs when children are unable to fall asleep without a certain object (e.g., pacifier, bottle) or situation (e.g., nursing, rocking).

21. What is the prevalence of sleep onset association disorder?

Approximately 15–20% of children, aged 6 months to 3 years, experience sleep-onset association disorder. After the age of 3 years, the prevalence significantly decreases. This disorder is relatively uncommon in adults.

22. What are sleep associations?

Sleep associations are conditions that are present at bedtime and usually required again after normal nighttime arousals. Positive sleep associations are those that the child can provide for himself or herself (e.g., thumbsucking, stuffed animal). Negative sleep associations require parental intervention (e.g., nursing, rocking) at bedtime and again after typical night wakings.

23. What happens if a child has sleep-onset association disorder?

Since sleep-onset associations are required to fall asleep at bedtime, when children arouse during the night, they need the same associations to return to sleep. If the association is not available (e.g., the mother is sleeping in a different room and unable to rock the child back to sleep), the result may be frequent and prolonged night wakings.

24. Do all children typically arouse during the night?

All children typically arouse on average 4–6 times during the night as a result of normal ultradian rhythms.

25. What is the difference between "self-soothers" and "signalers"?

Self-soothers are children who are able to soothe themselves back to sleep without parental intervention (e.g., breastfeeding, rocking) following a normal nighttime arousal. Signalers are children who alert their parents when they awaken by crying or going into the parents' room.

26. Do certain situations result in more frequent arousals or night wakings?

Yes. Children who share a room or bed with their parent(s), also called cosleeping, have been found to be more likely to awaken during the night and seek interaction with a parent. Babies who are breast-fed need to be fed more frequently and are also more likely to be nursed to sleep (a negative sleep association). Normal developmental milestones coincide with increased night wakings, especially between 9 and 12 months of age. Illnesses, vacations, and schedule changes can result in sleep disruptions and increased night wakings. Finally, colic or other medical conditions often result in more frequent arousals and typically require parental intervention.

27. When should a child be referred for treatment of sleep-onset association disorder?

When a child has difficulty in falling asleep at bedtime and/or returning to sleep during the night without parental intervention and this problem is highly disruptive to the family, the child should be referred to a sleep or mental health specialist who can address behavioral changes for the negative sleep associations.

28. What is the first step in helping a child learn to self-soothe?

It is important for children to learn to fall asleep at bedtime without parental intervention. This goal can be accomplished by putting the child to bed drowsy but awake. Once the child learns to fall asleep at bedtime on his or her own, this patterns will generalize to falling back to sleep after normal nighttime arousals.

29. What should parents do if the child cries when they put the child to bed drowsy but awake?

The different approaches to responding to a child's cries at bedtime include extinction ("crying it out"), graduated extinction, and scheduled fading of parental involvement.

30. What is extinction?

Extinction is based on operant theory: if you do not give attention or reinforce a certain behavior (e.g., crying), the behavior will decrease over time and eventually be eliminated. In terms of falling asleep, this approach translates into ignoring a child's cries until he or she falls asleep.

31. What challenges are associated with extinction?

The biggest challenge is that parents must be consistent and not respond to the child, no matter how long the child cries. If the parent "gives in" after a certain amount of time, the child learns simply to cry longer the next time, knowing that eventually he or she will get the desired response (e.g., parental intervention).

32. Will parents cause long-term psychological harm by letting their child "cry it out"?

No. Recent studies do not indicate any long-term psychological harm of "crying it out." Rather, extinction has been shown to be a successful intervention if it is done consistently. When properly used, extinction procedures typically show results in 3-5 days.

33. What is graduated extinction?

Graduated extinction involves putting the child to bed drowsy but awake and then ignoring the child's cries or requests for progressively longer periods of time (e.g., 2, 5, 10 minutes). Parents are more likely to follow through with graduated extinction, and it has been shown to be an effective intervention, taking several days to a few weeks to implement.

34. What if parents are unable to tolerate either extinction or graduated extinction?

Another alternative is scheduled fading of parental involvement as the child falls asleep. Four primary areas can be faded: (1) the amount of physical contact that the parent has with the child (e.g., holding, patting on back); (2) how close the parent is to the child (e.g., moving a chair two feet from the child's bed every two nights); (3) the amount of time between parental checks on the child; and (4) how long the parent spends in the room while checking on the child.

35. What is an extinction burst?

An extinction burst is an increase and intensification in a symptom (e.g., crying) that should be expected on the second night of any intervention. If parents are not warned about extinction bursts, they often become frustrated and noncompliant with intervention recommendations.

36. What other potential problems should be discussed with parents using extinction or

graduated extinction approaches to treat sleep-onset association disorder?

The child may become so upset that he or she vomits or cry so loud that a sibling is awakened. If parents are aware that these behaviors may occur, they are more likely to comply with treatment recommendations.

37. Do nighttime feedings help children sleep?

After children reach 6 months of age, they typically no longer require nighttime feedings. No evidence indicates that night feedings improve sleep quality or sleep quantity. In fact, the need for feeding during the night can become a learned behavior ("learned hunger"), which results in increased night wakings.

38. What is the prognosis for children with sleep-onset association disorder?

Without intervention, frequent and persistent night wakings are likely to continue. However, negative sleep associations tend to taper as children get older since many behaviors and situations decrease in frequency (e.g., nursing, rocking, bottles/pacifiers). With appropriate behavioral interventions, negative sleep associations can be reduced or eliminated, resulting in the child's ability to fall asleep on his or her own at bedtime as well as return to sleep following typical nighttime arousals.

BIBLIOGRAPHY

1. American Academy of Sleep Medicine: The International Classification of Sleep Disorders: Diagnostic and Coding Manual Revised. Westchester, IL, American Academy of Sleep Medicine, 1997.
2. Ferber R: Solve Your Child's Sleep Problems. New York, Simon & Schuster, 1985.
3. Goodlin-Jones BL, Burnham MM, Gaylor EE, Anders TF: Night waking, sleep-wake organization, and self-soothing in the first year of life. J Devel Behav Pediatr 22:226–233, 2001.
4. Kuhn BR, Elliott AJ: Treatment efficacy in behavioral pediatric sleep medicine. In Perlis ML, Lichstein KL (eds): Treating Sleep Disorders: Principles and Practice of Behavioral Sleep Medicine. New York, Jossey-Bass, 2003.
5. Kuhn BR, Weidinger D: Interventions for infant and toddler sleep disturbance: A review. Child Fam Behav Ther 22:33–50, 2000.
6. Lewin DS: Childhood insomnias: Limit setting and sleep onset association disorder: Diagnostic issues, behavioral treatment, and future directions. In Perlis ML, Lichstein KL (eds): Treating Sleep Disorders: Principles and Practice of Behavioral Sleep Medicine. New York, Jossey-Bass, 2003.
7. Mindell JA: Sleeping Through the Night: How Infants, Toddlers and Their Parents Can Get a Good Night's Sleep. New York, Harper Collins, 1997.
8. Mindell JA: Empirically supported treatments in pediatric psychology: Bedtime refusal and night wakings in young children. J Pediatr Psychol 24:465–481, 1999.
9. Mindell JA, Owens JA: A Clinical Guide to Pediatric Sleep: Diagnosis and Management of Sleep Problems. Philadelphia, Lippincott Williams & Wilkins, 2003.
10. Owens JL, France KG, Wiggs L: Behavioural and cognitive interventions for sleep disorders in infants and children: A review. Sleep Med Rev 3:281–302, 1999.
11. Reid MJ, Walter AL, O'Leary SG: Treatment of young children's bedtime refusal and nighttime wakings: A comparison of "standard" and graduated ignoring procedures. J Abnorm Child Psychol 27:5–16, 1999.

23. PEDIATRIC PARTIAL AROUSAL PARASOMNIAS

Lisa J. Meltzer, PhD, and Jodi A. Mindell, PhD

1. What are partial arousal parasomnias?

Partial arousal parasomnias are episodic sleep disorders, including sleep terrors and sleepwalking, that typically occur within 1–2 hours of falling asleep, last from a few minutes to 1 hour, and are characterized by retrograde amnesia. During these episodes, children and adolescents appear to be awake and do not respond to comforting by parents.

2. During what sleep stages do partial arousal parasomnias occur?

Sleep terrors and sleepwalking occur almost exclusively during slow-wave sleep (stages III and IV of non-REM sleep), and do not involve dreaming.

3. Is there a genetic component to partial arousal parasomnias?

Yes. There is an 80–90% chance that a child with sleep terrors or sleepwalking has an affected first-degree relative.

4. Are sleep terrors and sleepwalking indicative of a psychological disorder or a history of psychological trauma or harm?

No. Partial arousal parasomnias are a physiologic phenomenon. Although they may be triggered by stress, these behaviors do not indicate a primary psychological disorder or psychological trauma or harm.

5. What are sleep terrors?

Sleep terrors, or night terrors, have a sudden onset and are dramatic events that can include extreme agitation, fright, and/or confusion. They often involve crying and/or screaming. Children may not recognize their parents during these episodes and are not comforted by parental intervention.

6. How often do sleep terrors occur?

Sleep terrors can occur infrequently or multiple times per night, depending on the child.

7. What do children remember about sleep terrors in the morning?

Nothing. The child is totally unaware of his or her behavior during the night and does not recall the episodes in the morning. Sleep terrors are more upsetting to watch than to experience and are not at all traumatic to the child.

8. What is the prevalence of sleep terrors?

Approximately 3% of children experience sleep terrors, with the occurrence highest during the preschool and elementary school years. Episodes tend to be more frequent with an earlier age at onset.

9. Do children outgrow sleep terrors?

Typically children outgrow sleep terrors by adolescence, but some people experience sleep terrors into adulthood.

10. What is sleepwalking?

Sleepwalking is a common and benign sleep behavior in which the eyes are usually open, but the child may appear confused or dazed, answer questions inappropriately, and may appear agitated.

11. How often do children sleepwalk?

Sleepwalking can range in occurrence from infrequently to every night.

12. What is the prevalence of sleepwalking?

Between 15 and 40% of children sleepwalk on at least one occasion, with 3–4% having frequent (weekly, monthly) episodes. Sleepwalking typically begins between 4 and 6 years of age, with peak incidence between 4 and 8 years of age. Approximately one-third of children continue to have sleepwalking episodes for 5 years, and 10% of children have episodes for 10 years.

13. Is there a relationship between sleep terrors and sleepwalking?

Due to the common genetic predisposition, 10% of children who sleepwalk also have sleep terrors.

14. What factors exacerbate parasomnias?

Sleep deprivation, irregular sleep schedules, fever and illness, medications (e.g., chloral hydrate), environmental triggers (e.g., different room, noisy environment), stress, and anxiety can each lead to a partial arousal parasomnia.

15. Are there any medical conditions in which partial arousal parasomnias are more common?

People with migraine headaches and Tourette's syndrome appear to be at risk for partial arousal parasomnias.

16. What is the impact of a partial arousal parasomnia on the child and family?

Sleep terrors and sleepwalking can interfere with a child's social interactions. He or she may limit participation in overnight visits at a friend's house or summer camp due to embarrassment. In addition, parents often experience increased anxiety about whether there is an underlying cause as well as concerns about the child's safety during the night.

17. What is the difference between a sleep terror and a nightmare?

Nightmares are bad dreams that occur during REM sleep, whereas night terrors are physiologic episodes that occur during slow-wave sleep. Thus sleep terrors typically occur in the first third of the night, whereas nightmares typically occur in the last third of the night. In addition, children have frequent and vivid memories of nightmares with no recollection of sleep terrors. Finally, children are comforted by others after a nightmare, whereas parental intervention can exacerbate sleep terror events.

18. How are partial arousal parasomnias managed?

The primary interventions are reassurance and education. Parents should be encouraged to provide safety in the home. This strategy includes the use of gates on doorways or staircases, locking outside doors and windows, proper lighting in the hallway, and removing objects that a child may trip on during the night. A bell can also be used to alert parents if a sleepwalker leaves his or her room. Proper sleep hygiene (adequate sleep and regular sleep-wake schedule) is also important in the prevention of sleep terrors and sleepwalking. Behavioral interventions should be used as necessary to manage behaviorally based night wakings or bedtime refusal that may contribute to sleep deprivation. Finally, parents should avoid interference during an episode and should not discuss episodes the following day (discussion may increase the child's anxiety).

19. Are medications indicated?

In certain cases when parasomnia episodes are frequent or severe or if there is a high risk of injury or violent behavior, treatment with medications may be indicated. Short-acting benzodiazapines are the primary pharmacologic agent. When given at bedtime, these medications suppress slow-wave sleep in the first third of the night, which decreases the chance of a parasomnia episode.

20. What are scheduled awakenings?

Scheduled awakenings are a behavioral technique that is effective in eliminating or reducing partial arousal parasomnias when episodes occur on a nightly basis. This treatment involves having the parents wake the child approximately 15–30 minutes before the first parasomnia episode typically occurs. Treatment typically lasts for 2–4 weeks and can be reinstituted if the episodes return.

21. What is the prognosis for children with partial arousal parasomnias?

Most children outgrow partial arousal parasomnias during childhood. By 8 years of age, 50% of children no longer experience parasomnias. At puberty, there is a significant decrease in slow-wave sleep; thus most cases spontaneously resolve during adolescence.

BIBLIOGRAPHY

1. American Academy of Sleep Medicine: The International Classification of Sleep Disorders: Diagnostic and Coding Manual Revised. Westchester, IL, American Academy of Sleep Medicine, 1997.
2. Kuhn BR, Elliott AJ: Treatment efficacy in behavioral pediatric sleep medicine. In Perlis ML, Lichstein KL (eds): Treating Sleep Disorders: Principles and Practice of Behavioral Sleep Medicine. New York, Jossey-Bass, 2003.
3. Mahowald MW, Schenck CH: Diagnosis and management of parasomnias. Clin Cornerstone 2: 48–57, 2000.
4. Mindell JA. Sleep disorders in children. Health Psychol 12:151–162, 1993.
5. Mindell JA, Owens JA: A Clinical Guide to Pediatric Sleep: Diagnosis and Management of Sleep Problems. Philadelphia, Lippincott Williams & Wilkins, 2003.
6. Rosen GM, Ferber R, Mahowald M: Evaluation of parasomnias in children. Clin Adolesc Psychiatr Clin North Am 5:601–616, 1996.

24. SLEEP-DISORDERED BREATHING, PRIMARY SNORING, AND SUDDEN INFANT DEATH SYNDROME

Jean Silvestri, MD, and Debra Weese-Mayer, MD

SLEEP-DISORDERED BREATHING

Epidemiology

1. How common is sleep-disordered breathing in children?

Since sleep-disordered breathing may include the spectrum from quiet snoring to severe sleep apnea/hypopnea syndrome (SAHS), the frequency of sleep-disordered breathing depends on the definition and methodologies used to describe the disorder. Snoring may occur in children of all ages. Snoring as reported by questionnaire has a prevalence of 3–12%. The prevalence of obstructive sleep apnea is 1–3%.

2. What are the risk factors for sleep-disordered breathing in children?

In the pediatric population the finding or history of enlarged tonsils and adenoids plays a significant role. In patients who have other risk factors, such as obesity, craniofacial abnormalities, or abnormal upper airway tone associated with neurologic disorders, enlarged tonsils and adenoids are always dealt with in addition to the child's underlying problem. Snoring is also associated with a family history of tonsillectomy and adenoidectomy, passive smoking, and frequent upper respiratory infections.

3. Is there a gender or ethnic difference in sleep-disordered breathing rates in children?

Although there are gender differences in adult obstructive sleep apnea, no definitive data regarding the role of gender are available for the pediatric population. Data suggest that obstructive sleep apnea may be more common among African-American than among Caucasian children.

Pathophysiology

4. How is sleep-disordered breathing different in children and adults?

1. Age at presentation: The peak age of presentation in children is from 2 to 6 years, although SAHS has been documented from infancy through adulthood.

2. Risk factors
- Although obesity is associated with SAHS in adults as well as children, SAHS may be found in both normal-weight children and children with decreased growth.
- Adenotonsillar hypertrophy is a major cause for obstructive sleep apnea in the pediatric population but not among adults.

3. Manifestations
- Even though children may have only brief or partial airway upper airway obstruction (as compared with complete SAHS in adults), gas exchange abnormalities with hypoxemia and hypercarbia are frequently observed. From normative data, any duration of obstruction is abnormal in children. No normative data are available for the definition of an abnormal respiratory disturbance index (RDI), as commonly used in adults; normative data throughout childhood are limited.
- Pediatric SAHS is a disorder of predominantly REM sleep. Children with SAHS have preserved sleep architecture, and obstructive apneas are less likely to result in cortical arousals as compared with adults.

4. Physiologic sequelae: Pulmonary hypertension and cor pulmonale can result from SAHS in children compared with both pulmonary and systemic hypertension in adults.

5. Behavioral sequelae
- Daytime somnolence as seen in adults is often difficult to distinguish from school-week behavior in an average adolescent.
- In younger children, hyperactivity, developmental delay, and poor school performance are found.

5. Describe the role of genetics in pediatric sleep-disordered breathing.

There is a familial tendency to SAHS and a higher rate of tonsillectomy and adenoidectomy among parents of children with SAHS. The role of genetics is an avenue for further research.

6. What is meant by adenoid facies?

Adenoid facies is typically found in a child who breathes through the mouth and consists of allergic shiners and a hyponasal voice.

Diagnosis and Classification

7. What part of the physical examination is especially relevant in children suspected of having sleep apnea?

It is important to examine vital signs, including weight, height, and blood pressure. Ideally, weight and height should be viewed in the context of prior data to determine whether the child has fallen or begun to fall off the growth curve. Attention should be directed to the child's behavior. A complete ear, nose, and throat examination is essential, noting nonspecific findings related to adenotonsillar hypertrophy such as mouth breathing, hyponasal speech, adenoidal facies, and nasal obstruction. The craniofacial exam is important to determine whether an underlying syndrome is present and whether specific features predispose a child to obstructive sleep apnea, such as small triangular chin, retroposition of the mandible, steep mandibular plane, high-arched palate, long oval-shaped face, long soft palate, or bifid uvula. Signs of right ventricular hypertrophy or pulmonary hypertension with an increased second heart sound or right ventricular heave are significant consequences of SAHS in children.

8. What is a normal apnea-hypopnea index (AHI) in children?

There are no normative data for AHI or RDI in children. From the limited studies of normative data in children, central apnea is common, especially central apnea preceded by a sigh. However, obstructive apnea is rare. Thus any obstruction is considered abnormal in children; as noted above, even partial (as well as complete) obstruction can be associated with gas exchange abnormalities.

Prognosis and Treatment

9. What are the behavioral consequences of sleep-disordered breathing in children?

Children with sleep-disordered breathing can have a spectrum of medical, behavioral, and neurologic sequelae. SAHS can result in failure to thrive, growth failure, nocturnal enuresis, and cor pulmonale. Attention disorders, memory and learning problems, school failure, developmental delay, aggressiveness, and hyperactivity have been described and continue to be characterized.

Studies have been confounded by the age range of patients and coexistent medical and respiratory disorders. A population-based, cross-sectional study of 3019 5-year-old children revealed 19% with parent-reported hyperactivity, 18% with inattention, 12% with aggressiveness, and 10% with daytime sleepiness. Symptoms of sleep-disordered breathing were found in 25% of children. Children with sleep-disordered breathing were significantly more likely to have daytime sleepiness and problem behaviors such as hyperactivity, inattention, and aggressiveness.

10. What are the treatment options in children with sleep-disordered breathing?

Tonsillectomy and adenoidectomy remain the mainstay of treatment for most children and are also considered an option even in the face of other underlying causes. Other treatment options depend on the cause of the sleep-disordered breathing.

- With craniofacial abnormalities surgical reconstruction is the ultimate goal, but there may be several steps leading to the final result and relief of obstruction.
- Medical treatment options are often temporary, such as a nasopharyngeal airway or nasal steroids, or difficult, such as weight loss in obese patients.
- If abnormalities persist after surgical intervention with tonsillectomy and adenoidectomy, noninvasive mask positive airway pressure ventilation is considered with either continuous positive airway pressure (CPAP) or bilevel positive airway pressure (BiPAP).
- In some cases, use of supplemental oxygen may be considered for obstructive sleep apnea, but this option must be initiated in a monitored environment to determine whether supplemental oxygen will alter respiratory drive and result in significant hypercapnia and prolonged apnea.
- If treatment options fail, a tracheostomy may be indicated. However, because of increased familiarity with the technique of noninvasive ventilation and better mask interfaces, tracheostomy is a last resort.
- The surgical option called uvulopalatoplasty, commonly performed in adults, is typically not recommended for children.

11. How should children with suspected sleep apnea who undergo tonsillectomy and/or adenoidectomy be managed postoperatively?

Severity of the findings from the preoperative polysomnographic study aid in determining which children are at greater risk for postoperative complications. In addition, factors such as young age (less than 3 years), presence of failure to thrive or obesity, cor pulmonale, craniofacial anomalies, and neuromuscular disease place a child at greater risk for postoperative complications. Such children should be monitored postoperatively for obstruction and oxyhemoglobin desaturation, most likely as a result of postoperative airway edema and residual anesthetic agents. For children with severe preoperative hypercarbia, it is essential to monitor carbon dioxide values, taking care to avoid rapid decreases with manual or mechanical hyperventilation.

12. Discuss the role of oral appliances in children with sleep-disordered breathing.

Oral appliances such as the mandibular advancement device are not typically used for children with sleep-disordered breathing because the mandible is still developing. However, in a study of children with SAHS accompanied by malocclusion, a personalized oral jaw-positioning device improved clinical symptoms as well as polysomnographic data. External nasal dilator strips have been studied only in a small group of infants with and without nasal congestion and have not been examined in older children. However, surgically implanted mandibular advancement devices have been used in children with craniofacial abnormalities with management by a team of reconstructive surgeons and dentists.

PRIMARY SNORING

Epidemiology

13. How common is snoring in children?

Questionnaires about snoring report a prevalence of 3–12%. Primary snoring is identified in the absence of apnea, hypoventilation, or excessive arousals.

14. Is snoring in children gender-related?

There does not appear to be a gender difference.

Pathophysiology

15. What are the health consequences of snoring in children?

Primary snoring is typically not associated with physiologic compromise and is considered a benign condition. The question is whether primary snoring progresses along a continuum to upper airway resistance syndrome or even obstructive sleep apnea, with a need to distinguish primary snoring from SAHS.

16. Discuss the natural history of primary snoring in children.

Data regarding the natural history of primary snoring in children are limited. One must account for age at identification and the impact of other associated risk factors, which may increase the risk for development of obstructive sleep apnea over time. Long-term studies are indicated to better understand the evolution of the entire disease spectrum and its consequences.

Diagnosis and Classification

17. How can the history help differentiate primary snoring from obstructive sleep apnea?

Unfortunately, it is difficult to identify from history, questionnaire, or tonsillar size alone whether snoring is just an "acoustic disturbance" or "physiologic compromise." In addition, without some form of monitoring, severity of physiologic compromise cannot be assessed.

18. Discuss the role of polysomnography in the diagnosis of primary snoring.

Polysomnography is considered the gold standard in identification of sleep-disordered breathing and obstructive sleep apnea. The American Academy of Pediatrics *Clinical Practice Guideline on the Diagnosis and Management of Childhood Obstructive Sleep Apnea Syndrome* states that "a diagnostic evaluation is useful in discriminating between primary snoring and SAHS with the gold standard being polysomnography." This resource may be of limited availability, but other types of monitoring, such as pulse oximetry, actigraphy, audio or video recordings, and multichannel recordings, in the hospital or at home, have not been extensively studied. It must be cautioned that an accurate diagnosis is necessary to determine appropriate treatment and to avoid unnecessary intervention; it is also essential to prevent sequelae due to repeated hypoxemia and hypercarbia.

Treatment

19. Does primary snoring always require treatment?

Primary snoring is a benign condition that does not require treatment. However, it does require physiologic evaluation in a pediatric respiratory physiology laboratory and careful follow-up to determine resolution or exacerbation.

SUDDEN INFANT DEATH SYNDROME

Epidemiology

20. How common is sudden infant death syndrome (SIDS)?

Although SIDS remains a leading cause of death during infancy (third behind congenital malformations and low birthweight), the incidence has declined worldwide over time. This decline is associated with the increased incidence of supine sleeping. The most recent SIDS rate from the United States is 0.56 deaths per 1000 live births in 2001; however, there is a persistent racial disparity in SIDS deaths. Although all racial groups demonstrate a reduction in SIDS deaths, in 2001 the SIDS rates in infants of African-American and American Indian mothers was more than double that of non-Hispanic Caucasian mothers.

21. What are the nonmodifiable risk factors for SIDS?

Characteristics of SIDS include a peak incidence at 2-4 months of age and an excess of deaths in male infants. Other risk factors include young maternal age, high parity, prematurity, low birth weight, and multiple births.

22. What are the modifiable risk factors for SIDS?

- The greatest impact has been in relation to infant sleep position. As more infants have been placed on their backs to sleep, the incidence of SIDS has decreased. Side position is not an acceptable alternative; this unstable position confers an increased risk because most infants will roll to the prone position.
- Immunizations reduce the risk of SIDS.
- Overheating has also been associated with an increased risk of SIDS and has the potential for modification.
- Both pre- and postnatal tobacco smoke exposure (by the mother as well as by any smokers in the vicinity of the pregnant mother or infant) increases the risk of SIDS. There is a direct correlation with hours of exposure and SIDS, but this factor may be difficult to modify.
- Soft bedding also confers an increased risk for SIDS.
- Bed sharing (mother in bed with the infant) is a risk behavior when the mother is a smoker or has consumed alcohol.
- Room sharing (parent in the room with the infant) reduces the risk of SIDS.

Pathophysiology

23. What is the "sleep and arousal hypothesis" regarding SIDS?

Data support a maturational response to arousal from hypoxia during sleep. Newborn infants and young infants have a strong hypoxic arousal response, most likely mediated by the developing brainstem. As infants enter the stage of increased risk of SIDS (2 months of age), this protective response is diminished. Thus it is appealing to view absent arousal response as an explanation for SIDS.

24. Why is sleep position thought to be important in this patient group?

Several studies have identified that infants who succumbed to SIDS were more likely to be placed to sleep and/or found in the prone position. Identification of the prone sleep position as a key risk factor in SIDS and implementation of aggressive "Back to Sleep" educational campaigns have led to the remarkable world-wide decrease in the SIDS incidence. It has also provided insights into possible mechanisms, such as altered thermal control in the prone position, increased vulnerability to rebreathing in the prone position, and altered arousal thresholds in the prone position. All of these potential mechanisms may have interactions with other risk factors such as sleep environment and smoking.

25. What is the role of respiratory control in infants with SIDS or their siblings?

Because of the inability to identify prospectively the infant who will die of SIDS, investigators have extensively studied respiratory control in healthy newborns to gain insights into an infant's potential vulnerability. The interaction between infant susceptibility, environmental stressors (e.g., sleep environment, tobacco exposure), and peak age of vulnerability (age 2-4 months) is known as the triple risk hypothesis. Studies of SIDS siblings have been limited and do not show distinct differences.

Diagnosis and Classification

26. What is meant by the terms *apparent life-threatening event* and *near miss* as they relate to SIDS?

An apparent life-threatening event (ALTE) has been defined as an event that is frightening to the observer and characterized by a combination of apnea, skin color change, marked change in muscle tone, choking, and gagging. These episodes were previously known as "near miss SIDS"; however, most infants survived and were not at increased risk of sudden death. This term has been abandoned since the NIH consensus statement in 1987. The ALTE definition is characterized by the caregiver's reaction to the event; thus, this interpretation may either increase or decrease the severity of the event.

27. How is an infant with ALTE evaluated?

The evaluation of an infant with an ALTE is directed at determining an underlying etiology. The work-up includes a period of observation and complete history and physical examination as well as directed laboratory investigations, which may include a multichannel recording or full polysomnography to determine whether the infant has an underlying problem of respiratory control. Typical ALTEs are the result of gastroesophogeal reflux, seizures, infection, cardiorespiratory problems, or metabolic disorders. Often no underlying etiology is found. In infants with recurrent ALTEs without an underlying etiology, one must consider induced or fabricated illness and use a multidisciplinary approach.

Prognosis and Treatment

28. What is the role of prevention in this patient group?

All infant caregivers should be counseled about avoidance of SIDS risk factors and maintaining a safe sleeping environment:

- Place the infant on his or her back to sleep.
- Use a firm sleeping surface without soft pillows, blankets, or crib toys.
- Maintain a smoke-free environment.
- Do not let the infant get too warm during sleep.
- The infant's head should remain uncovered.

29. What other treatment modalities are available?

Recent genetic evidence has implicated the serotonergic system as a cause of SIDS. Decreased serotonergic receptor binding has been found in the arcuate nucleus of SIDS cases compared with controls. A recent U.S. study including 46 Caucasian and 44 African-American SIDS cases found an excess of the long (L) allele and L/L genotype in the promoter region of the serotonin transporter gene (5-HTT) in the SIDS group compared with controls, and fewer SIDS cases were documented with the short allele. In addition, investigation of the 5-HTT intron 2 polymorphism in the same 90 cases of SIDS revealed that the intron 2 polymorphism is associated with SIDS and that the 12 repeat allele and the L12 haplotypes are significantly associated with SIDS, primarily in the African-American population. These findings open many avenues of future research and offer the potential for interventional strategies as well as risk assessment for appropriate counseling of families.

BIBLIOGRAPHY

1. American Thoracic Society: Standards and indications for cardiorespiratory sleep studies in children. Am J Respir Crit Care Med 153:866–878, 1996.
2. American Academy of Pediatrics, Section on Pediatric Pulmonology, Subcommittee on Obstructive Sleep Apnea Syndrome: Clinical practice guideline: Diagnosis and management of childhood obstructive sleep apnea syndrome. Pediatrics 109:704–712, 2002.
3. Arias E, MacDorman MF, Strobino DM, Guyer B: Annual summary of vital statistics—2002. Pediatrics 112(6):1215–1230, 2003.
4. Fleming PJ, Blair P, Sawczenko A: Sudden infant death syndrome: Modifiable risk factors and the window of vulnerability. In Loughlin GM, Carroll JL, Marcus CL (eds): Sleep and Breathing in Children: A Developmental Approach. New York, Marcel Dekker, 2000, pp 443–464.
5. Gottlieb DJ, Vezina RM, Chase C, et al: Symptoms of sleep-disordered breathing in 5-year-old children are associated with sleepiness and problem behaviors. Pediatrics 112:870–877, 2003.

6. Marcus CL, Omlin KJ, Basinski DJ, Bailey SL, Rachal AB, VonPechmann WS, Keens TG, Ward SL. Normal polysomnogram values for children and adolescents. Am Rev Respir Dis 146: 1235–1239, 1992.
7. Marcus CL: Sleep disordered breathing in children. Am J Respir Crit Care Med 164:16–30, 2001.
8. Panigrahy A, Filiano J, Sleeper LA, et al: Decreased serotonin receptor binding in rhombic lip derived regions of the medulla oblongata in the sudden infant death syndrome. J Neuropathol Exp Neurol 59:377–384, 2000.
9. Redline S, Tishler PV, Hans MG, et al: Racial differences in sleep-disordered breathing in African-Americans and Caucasians. Am J Respir Crit Care Med 155:186–192, 1997.
10. Rosen GM, Muckle RP, Mahowald MW, et al: Postoperative respiratory compromise in children with obstructive sleep apnea syndrome: Can it be anticipated? Pediatrics 93:784–788, 1994.
11. Waters KA, Everwtt FM, Bruderer JW, Sullivan CE: Obstructive sleep apnea: The use of nasal CPAP in 80 children. Am J Respir Crit Care Med 152:780–785, 1995.
12. Weese-Mayer DE, Zhou L, Berry-Kravis EM, et al: Association of the serotonin transporter gene with sudden infant death syndrome: A haplotype analysis. Am J Med Genet 122A:238–245, 2003.
13. Weese-Mayer DE, Berry-Kravis EM, Maher BS, et al: Sudden infant death syndrome: Association with a promoter polymorphism of the serotonin transporter gene. Am J Med Genet 117A: 268–274, 2003.

25. PEDIATRIC SLEEP AND MEDICAL DISORDERS

Mark Splaingard, MD

ENURESIS

1. What is the difference between nocturnal enuresis and sleep-related enuresis?

Nocturnal enuresis is involuntary voiding during nighttme sleep at an age when volitional control of micturition is expected. Most authorities agree that 5 years of age is the developmental level when concerns and interventions over bedwetting begin to become appropriate. **Sleep-related enuresis** (SRE) is the preferred term to describe bedwetting during sleep at anytime (not just at night).

2. How common is sleep-related enuresis?

SRE has a declining prevalence with increasing age. The incidence is approximately 30% of 4-year-olds, 15% of 5-year-olds, and 10% of 6-year-olds, with a spontaneous remission rate of approximately 15% for each year afterward. About 3% of 12-year-olds and 1% of 15-year-olds remain affected. The frequency among adults is probably less than 1%. There is a familial predisposition, with the highest incidence (75%) in children whose parents were both enuretic in childhood.

3. Distinguish between primary and secondary sleep-related enuresis.

SRE is termed **primary** when the child has not had a period of more than 3 months of sleep continence since birth. SRE is termed **secondary** when it redevelops in a child who formerly was continuously "dry" during sleep for at least 3 months.

4. Does primary or secondary enuresis have a better prognosis? Why?

Primary enuresis has a higher rate of spontaneous remission then secondary enuresis. Organic or psychological factors appear to be more common in children with secondary enuresis. Children who develop secondary enuresis should be carefully evaluated for new-onset obstructive sleep apnea, diabetes insipidus, diabetes mellitus, renal disease, nocturnal seizures, spinal cord tumors, and urinary tract infections based on signs and symptoms outlined in the table below. An organic cause is identified in about 5% of children with SRE. A careful psychological history should be pursued in all children with secondary enuresis. Although psychological causes are rare (< 1%) in primary SRE, they are common in secondary SRE. Abuse and neglect, situational stress, separation from parents, anxiety, and birth of a sibling have been associated with secondary SRE. When an identifiable cause for enuresis cannot be found, the symptom is termed *functional* (a polite term to cloak our ignorance)

Signs and Symptoms That Should Raise Suspicion of an Organic Cause of Enuresis

Signs	
Enlarged tonsils	Abnormal neurologic examination
Craniofacial abnormalities	Pes cavus (high-arched feet)
Abnormal genital examination	Sacral hair tuft or dimple

Symptoms	
	Polydipsia
Dyspnea	Seizures
Hematuria	

Table continued on next page

Signs and Symptoms That Should Raise Suspicion of an Organic Cause of Enuresis (continued)

Hesitancy	Lower back pain
Urgency	Severe snoring
Frequency	Prior urinary tract infection
Polyuria	History of genitourinary surgery
Polyphagia	Daytime enuresis

5. Describe the two patterns of SRE. Which is more common?

SRE is classified into two patterns. **Monosymptomatic** enuresis is characterized by involuntary voiding during asleep without daytime symptoms or other symptoms referred to the urogenital tract. **Polysymptomatic** enuresis is associated with bladder symptoms such as urinary urgency, frequency, and voiding dysfunction. Eighty-five percent of children with SRE have monosynaptic enuresis.

6. When does SRE generally occur at night?

Polysomnographic evaluations have shown that enuresis usually occurs during the first half of the night during non–rapid-eye-movement (NREM) sleep. Enuresis is considered as a disorder of arousal, with elevated sleep arousal threshold and inability of enuretic children to awaken during episodes of bedwetting. Several studies have demonstrated elevated sleep arousal thresholds in response to auditory stimuli in children with SRE and an increased depth of delta sleep during computerized electroencephalographic (EEG) analysis. However, the sleep architecture (length, organization, and morphology of sleep stages) does not appear substantially different between enuretic and nonenuretic children.

7. What is the exact mechanism of nocturnal enuresis in children?

The exact mechanism explaining the symptoms of enuresis has not been discovered. A three-system etiologic model has been proposed: (1) lack of vasopressin during sleep, (2) bladder instability, and (3) defective arousal mechanisms from sleep.

8. How is enuresis treated?

Children with primary or monosymptomatic enuresis may respond to nonpharmacologic therapies (e.g., behavior modifications and operant conditioning devices with noise at the time bedwetting occurs), and these treatments should be considered first. Nonpharmacologic interventions can result in remission rates of 50–70%. Treatments with tricyclic antidepressants (TCAs) result in a remission rate of 10–40%. Imipramine and other TCAs have been shown to be effective in the treatment of enuresis at relatively low doses of 10–75 mg/day. Response tends to be rapid, occurring within the first 3–4 days at an appropriate dose. In most cases, symptoms reappear after the drug is withdrawn. The development of tolerance to antidepressants is common and requires an increase in dosage. Antidepressants should not be continued indefinitely because enuresis may remit spontaneously. Oral administration at bedtime of desmopressin (DDAVP), a synthetic analog of antidiuretic hormone (ADH), stops bedwetting in 60–75% of children. Response is rapid, often within 1 week.

ASTHMA

9. Discuss the relationship of bronchial asthma to sleep disruption in children.

Asthma is a reversible obstructive lung disease manifesting as recurrent coughing, wheezing, and dyspnea in response to environmental triggers. Surveys indicate that asthma prevalence rates in children range from 5% to 15%. Significant worsening in lung functioning during the nighttime in children with asthma may be due to a combination of factors related to sleep or circadian events, as shown in the table below.

At least 1 awakening at night occurs in 34% of children with mild-to-moderate asthma, and 14% have 3 or more awakenings at night. Asthmatic children have more frequent arousals, increased wake time, decreased mean sleep time, and marked reduction of stage 4 (slow-wave) sleep. These changes in sleep architecture correlate with asthma severity indices. Poor sleeping patterns in children with nocturnal asthma can result in significant daytime consequences, including poor school performance, attention problems, and neurocognitive dysfunction.

Factors Contributing to Worsening of Asthma During Sleep

- Increase in airway resistance
- Decrease in lung volume
- Enhanced airway inflammation
- Nocturnal gastroesophageal reflux
- Increased pulmonary capillary blood volume
- Reduced mucociliary clearance

10. When do healthy children have their lowest peak expiratory flow rate?

Healthy children show a circadian variation in peak expiratory flow rate that reaches a nadir around 4:00 AM. The amplitude of this circadian change is much greater in asthmatics. Similar variations have been identified in the cutaneous immediate hypersensitivity response to house dust allergens and in airway inflammation, as documented by increase in inflammatory cells in the bronchoalveolar lavage fluid of patients with nocturnal asthma. The temporal relationships between individual sleep stages and pulmonary function are inconsistent. The hour of the morning appears more critical for drop in flows than a particular stage of sleep.

11. What factors contributing to nocturnal asthma may complicate the treatment of children?

Contributing factors for nocturnal asthma include allergic rhinitis, rhinosinusitis, and environmental allergies to indoor pets. Gastroesophageal reflux has been reported in a high percentage of children with nocturnal asthma; vagally mediated reflex bronchoconstriction is induced by esophageal acid and microaspiration. Treatment for nocturnal asthma symptoms includes treatment of contributory factors, adequate doses of anti-inflammatory therapy, long-acting inhaled beta agonists once or twice daily, or sustained-release theophylline once a day. Administration of oral corticosteroids in the evening appears to be more effective in controlling nocturnal symptoms in patients with steroid-dependent asthma.

CYSTIC FIBROSIS

12. What sleep problems are associated with cystic fibrosis (CF)?

Frequent coughing may cause significant sleep disruption in patients with CF. Oxygen desaturation at night can be a major problem in patients with moderate or severe cystic fibrosis, defined as a forced expiratory volume in one second (FEV_1) < 65% of the predicted value. Sleep apnea-hypopnea syndrome (SAHS) is rarely responsible for oxygen desaturation in patients with CF over 7 years of age. The exact mechanism leading to desaturation is probably a combination of hypoventilation caused by changes in mechanics of breathing due to de-recruitment of ventilatory muscles and ventilation-perfusion mismatching due to reduction in functional residual capacity during sleep.

13. What sleep stage is generally associated with the worst oxygen desaturation in patients with CF?

Oxygen desaturation is usually worse in patients with CF during REM sleep due to paralysis of all respiratory muscles except the diaphragms.

14. What daytime factors predict when patients with CF are likely to have nocturnal oxygen desaturation?

Nocturnal pulse oximetry studies may be abnormal in patients with moderate lung disease, even when awake resting oxygen saturation is normal. Studies have shown that an FEV_1 < 65% and a resting oxygen saturation (while sitting awake) < 94% are risk factors for oxygen desaturation at night. One study found that 40% of such patients had oxygen saturation < 90% for > 5% of sleep time.

15. What is the treatment for oxygen desaturation at night in patients with CF?

Addition of supplemental oxygen in patients with CF improves some daytime symptoms but does not lead to improved survival. Nocturnal oxygen therapy improves oxygenation during sleep but usually with accompanying increase in arterial partial pressure of carbon dioxide (pCO_2). Bilevel positive airway pressure support (BiPAP) with or without oxygen prevents hypoventilation during REM sleep and secondary oxygen desaturation. Overcoming REM-related hypoventilation with use of BiPAP may be important in delaying the onset of awake hypoxemia and hypercapnia, both of which are markers for poor prognosis.

CRANIOFACIAL ABNORMALITIES

16. What sleep-related problems occur in children with congenital craniofacial abnormalities?

Sleep-disordered breathing is described in infants and children with Pierre Robin sequence, Goldenhar's syndrome, trisomy 21, Treacher Collins syndrome, and velocardiofacial syndrome. It is also reported in children with cleft lips and palate who have undergone secondary corrective surgery to decrease nasal airflow and improve speech. Most problems are related to respiratory disturbances caused by upper airway obstruction.

17. What is pharyngeal flap surgery? What are the risks of this procedure?

A pharyngeal flap is a surgical treatment for marked nasalization of speech seen in some children with cleft palate after primary palatoplasty or in children with velopharyngeal insufficiency, which is abnormal nasopharyngeal closure that can compromise speech. The objective of pharyngeal flap surgery is to decrease the size of the velopharyngeal opening by placement of a soft tissue flap elevated from the posterior pharyngeal wall between the wall and the velum or palate. Flap surgery significantly reduces the size of the velopharynx to the point that nasal respiration is sometimes compromised during sleep and exercise. Most of these patients snore and occasionally have obstructive symptoms during sleep.

Obstructive apnea has been observed in up to 90% of patients 2–3 days after pharyngeal flap surgery. By 3–4 months after surgery, however, the frequency of obstructive events had returned toward baseline and was within normal limits in 80% of children.

18. What is the treatment for airway compromise after pharyngeal flap surgery?

After pharyngeal flap surgery, children occasionally have nasal airway obstruction sufficiently severe to warrant surgical revision or takedown of the flap. Nasal continuous positive airway pressure (CPAP) has been used both in the immediate postoperative period and for prolonged upper airway obstruction. Older children may recover from sleep apnea-hypopnea syndrome (SAHS) with growth as reconfiguration of the mandible and soft tissues proceed during adolescence. Many surgeons stress the value of managing obstructive symptoms at night with CPAP, if technically possible, until facial bone development can occur.

19. What is Pierre Robin sequence?

Pierre Robin sequence is a congenital anomaly that includes micrognathia, glossoptosis (abnormally placed tongue), and cleft palate. Because of the micrognathia the tongue tends to roll back into the throat and may be sucked into the pharynx or trapped in the cleft palate during breathing or swallowing. This problem occurs especially when the child is in the supine position. The affected child may present with noisy breathing, snoring, stridor, cyanosis, difficult feeding, or aspiration pneumonia.

20. How is Pierre Robin sequence treated?

Airway obstruction in children with Pierre Robin sequence can be treated with a variety of methods based on severity of obstruction. Nonsurgical interventions include adoption of the prone position, insertion of a nasopharyngeal tube, tongue/lip adhesion procedure, and tracheal intubation. Surgical interventions include mandibular distraction (see Figs. 1–3) or tracheostomies. Prone positioning works in approximately 70% of cases. The position is maintained for 5–6 months until the patient can undergo surgery.

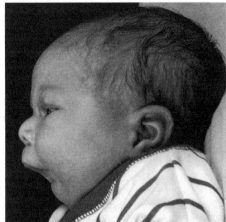

Figure 1. Infant with Pierre Robin sequence at 10 days.

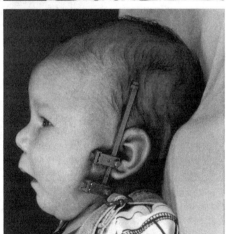

Figure 2. Same infant at 21 days of age with left mandibular distraction in place.

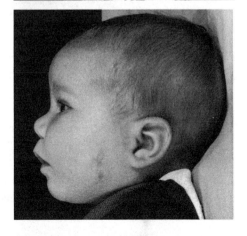

Figure 3. Same infant at 3 months of age 6 weeks after mandibular distraction removed. (All photographs from Denny A, Kalantarian B: Mandibular distraction in neonates: A strategy to avoid tracheostomy. Plast Reconstr Surg 109:896–904, 2002, with permission of The Children's Hospital of Wisconsin.)

GASTROESOPHAGEAL REFLUX

21. What is the incidence of gastroesophageal reflux in infants and children?

Gastroesophageal reflux (GER), the passage of gastric contents into the esophagus, is a normal physiologic process that occurs in all age groups. A pediatric practice-based survey estimated that vomiting, a common symptom of GER, is noted in 50% of infants in the first 3 months of life, in 67% of 4-month-old infants, and in 5% of 10- to 12-month-old infants.

22. What is gastroesophageal reflux disease?

Gastroesophageal reflux disease (GERD) is associated with symptoms that include feeding difficulties, failure to thrive, and recurrent respiratory symptoms. Transient, vagally mediated relaxations of the lower esophageal sphincter appear to be the main mechanism for GER and are not related to weak lower esophageal sphincter pressure.

23. How does sleep affect gastroesophageal physiology?

Sleep has significant influence on the physiology of upper gastrointestinal tract, as shown in the table below. A circadian rhythm of gastric acid secretion has been demonstrated, with peaks between 9:00 PM and midnight. During sleep children with GER may be at risk to develop esophageal pain and sleep disturbances. Sleep appears to be a vulnerable time for children with GER, and alteration of clearance mechanisms may predispose patients to serious complications such as esophagitis. Sleep-related GER may also lead to extra-esophageal complications, including stridor, chronic cough, and recurrent wheezing. However, children have higher arousal threshold in sleep, making it less likely for children with GER to have sleep disturbances as significant as those in adults.

Sleep-related Risk Factors for Gastroesophageal Reflux

* Increased arousals/awakenings
* Reduced swallow frequency
* Decreased salivary secretion
* Fall in upper esophageal sphincter (UES) tone
* Supine positioning
* Prolonged acid clearance time

24. What is the relationship between gastroesophageal reflux, apnea of prematurity, and apparent life-threatening events?

Protective airway reflexes, including laryngeal chemoreflex and esophagolaryngeal reflexes, are possible mechanisms for airway closure associated with reflux events in infants with apena of prematurity (AOP) and apparent life-threatening events (ALTEs). Although this association is intellectually appealing, simultaneously performed polysomnographic studies with pH monitoring have generally failed to identify any temporal association between the apneic events and reflux episodes in most infants with ALTE. However, individual children may be affected. Nonacid reflux, diagnosed by esophageal impedance, has recently been proposed as a possible mechanism of apnea, but this theory requires verification.

25. What is the treatment of nocturnal gastroesophageal reflux in children?

Limited data are available about the use of prokinetic agents and acid-suppressive therapies in children with nocturnal GER. A therapeutic trial may be justified in the uncomfortable child with sleep maintenance insomnia and suspected GERD. Although prone positioning has been shown to be effective in reducing the severity of GER, supine positioning confers the lowest risk for sudden infant death syndrome (SIDS) in infants under 12 months of age and is recommended by the American Academy of Pediatrics.

DOWN SYNDROME

26. What sleep state differences are seen in children with Down syndrome compared with normal children?

Down syndrome, the single most common genetic cause of mental retardation, is due to either an extra chromosome 21 (trisomy 21) or translocation of the q22 segment of chromosome 21 to another chromosome, which accounts for 4% of cases. In one study, sleep transition from perinatal to infantile patterns, as measured by disappearance of the trace alterant (TA) pattern, occurred later in infants with Down syndrome compared with controls (55 vs. 33 days). Sleep spindles appeared later and were less abundant throughout the first year of life in infants with Down syndrome. This pattern is similar to congenital hypothyroidism, suggesting a relationship between development of sleep spindles and brain maturation. The number of REM periods and eye movements during REM sleep is decreased in Down syndrome, with a longer REM latency (time from sleep onset to beginning of REM sleep) compared with normal children. A reduced percentage of REM sleep has been associated with lower IQ in children with Down syndrome.

27. What is the prevalence of sleep-related upper airway obstruction in children with Down syndrome?

The prevalence of sleep-related upper airway obstruction in Down syndrome is between 30% and 60%. Age, obesity, and presence of congenital heart disease do not affect the incidence.

28. What anatomic abnormalities are associated with sleep-related breathing problems in Down syndrome?

Children with Down syndrome may have midfacial and mandibular hypoplasia, narrow palate, glossoptosis (abnormal tongue size and position), reduced pharyngeal tone, prominent adenoids/ tonsils, laryngotracheal abnormalities, hypothyroidism, and obesity. Diminished hypoxic drive may contribute to centrally mediated apnea, hypoventilation, and respiratory failure. Congenital heart disease, including atrial and ventricular septal defects, can enhance the development of pulmonary arterial hypertension by causing left-to-right shunts and increased pulmonary blood flow. Pulmonary arterial hypertension and cor pulmonale can also occur in infants with Down syndrome without congenital heart disease due to reduction in pulmonary vascular surface area and peripheral extension of arterial smooth muscle, causing increased reactivity of pulmonary vessels to hypoxia and acidosis. Cheyne-Stokes respiration, hypoventilation, and cor pulmonale due to SAHS have been associated with unexplained pulmonary hypertension in patients with Down syndrome.

29. Discuss the site of airway obstruction in Down syndrome. How is it evaluated?

Airway patency in Down syndrome may be compromised at several sites, thereby reducing airway caliber. Traditional methods to evaluate the upper airway in children with Down syndrome include plain lateral neck x-rays, cephalometric measurements, airway fluoroscopy, and nasopharyngoscopy. Modern imaging techniques such as computer tomography (CT) scans and magnetic resonance imaging (MRI) provide more comprehensive anatomic details. MRI imaging of the upper airway in children with Down syndrome without SAHS does not show increased adenoidal or tonsillar volume. Reduced upper airway size is caused by soft tissue encroachment within a smaller mid and lower facial skeleton.

30. Discuss the treatment for upper airway obstruction in children with Down syndrome.

The selection of appropriate therapy for upper airway obstruction in children with Down syndrome is influenced by the anatomic structure of the individual child. Use of routine adenoidectomy and tonsillectomy is controversial because this approach fails to improve drooling or tongue protrusion and can result in hypernasality. Tonsillectomy and adenoidectomy alone infrequently provide long-lasting relief of obstruction. Surgical treatments involving soft tissue and skeletal alterations include tongue reduction, tongue hyoid advancement, uvulopalatopharyngoplasty, and maxillary midfacial advancement. Occasionally, children require tracheostomies. Nonsurgical treatments that may be appropriate in these patients include weight loss protocols, control of sinusitis or nasal allergies, and the use of CPAP or BiPAP during sleep.

SICKLE CELL DISEASE

31. What problems may be found during sleep in children with sickle cell disease?

Sickle cell disease (SCD) is one of the common beta-chain hemoglobinopathies, characterized by chronic hemolytic anemia and vaso-occlusive crisis related to the production of abnormal hemoglobin. Repeated vaso-occlusive crises can lead to multiple organ dysfunction, including acute chest syndrome, chronic lung disease, and cerebrovascular disease. Hypoxemia has been suggested as a risk factor for vaso-occlusive pain crises since polymerization of deoxygenated sickle hemoglobin is the primary molecular event in the pathogenesis of SCD. Episodic and continuous nocturnal hypoxemia is common and has been described in up to 40% of children with SCD. Two mechanisms of nocturnal hypoxemia include SAHS secondary to adenotonsillar hypertrophy and SCD-related chronic lung disease. Extramedullary hematopoiesis and repeated infections are possible causes for tonsillar and adenoidal hypertrophy.

32. What is the prevalence of obstructive sleep apnea in children with sickle cell disease?

The estimated prevalence of SAHS in SCD is 30–40%. Baseline hypoxemia during sleep occurs in 10–15% of children with a median age of 7–8 years.

33. Describe the management of children with SCD and suspected upper airway obstruction.

Screening and appropriate management of nocturnal hypoxemia have been recommended for primary prevention of central nervous system events in children with sickle cell disease. Although a clear causal relationship between hypoxemia due to SAHS and severity of vaso-occlusive episodes is not universally accepted, it seems prudent to evaluate symptomatic patients with SCD for SAHS and nocturnal hypoxemia by polysomnographic studies. Adenotonsillectomy may improve symptoms of snoring and eliminate hypoxemic episodes in patients with SAHS. Children with SCD are at higher risk, however, than control patients for postoperative complications after adenotonsillectomy. Preoperative transfusion prior to adenotonsillectomy to maintain a minimum hematocrit of 35% has been recommended. Currently no data support the use of continuous nocturnal supplemental oxygen to prevent vaso-occlusive episodes in patients with SCD and nocturnal hypoxemia.

OBESITY

34. How is obesity defined in children? How common is it?

Body mass index (BMI) varies with age and gender, and its use is relatively new in pediatric medicine. Children with a BMI > 95th percentile for age and sex or > 30 kg/m^2 are considered overweight. Using this definition, the prevalence of overweight children in the United States in the current decade is 15.3% among 6- to 11-year-olds and 10.4% among 2- to 5-year-olds. The prevalence of obesity is even higher in low-income families and minorities. In adults, a BMI > 25 is defined as overweight and a BMI > 30 defines obesity. By these standards, 30% of American adults are obese.

35. What is the incidence of SAHS in obese children?

In one study, 46% of overweight children with an average weight 184% of ideal body weight without sleep complaints had abnormal polysomnograms. One study reported that 37% of snoring overweight adolescents had abnormal polysomnograms, with 5% of the patients requiring clinical interventions. A correlation has been detected between the degree of insulin resistance in obese children and the severity of sleep-disordered breathing.

36. Discuss the quality of life of children with obesity and SAHS.

Children with obesity and SAHS were found to have poorer performance on standardized neurocognitive tests than obese children without SAHS. The severity of SAHS, as measured by total number of apneic and hypopneic episodes, was significantly correlated to the severity of neurocognitive impairments. Shockingly, in one study obese children with SAHS reported significantly lower health-related quality of life scores than obese children without SAHS and scores similar to those of children diagnosed with cancer.

37. Discuss the treatment of SAHS in an obese child.

Treatment of SAHS in obese children is multidisciplinary and challenging. Moderate weight loss in obese adults with SAHS often improves oxygenation during both sleep and wakefulness, decreases the collapsibility of the nasopharynx, and decreases the number of breathing events. Studies in children are lacking, but weight reduction probably has similar benefits. Successful weight loss and maintenance have been reported in less than 5% of obese adult patients. Although there are a few reports of long-term successful weight-reduction programs in childhood obesity, many children experiencing respiratory difficulties cannot adhere to diet restriction or resume physical activities essential for weight loss. Ear, nose, and throat (ENT) evaluation for potential correction of nasopharyngeal abnormalities, including tonsillar hypertrophy, deviation of nasal septum, and adenoidal hypertrophy, is essential in all children with obesity and SAHS. However, long-term improvement is complicated by the finding that tonsillectomy with or without adenoidectomy is associated with a subsequent increase in BMI in the next year in both obese and morbidly obese children. Some obese children remain obstructed even after adenoidectomy/tonsillectomy. CPAP may be useful in obese and morbidly obese children with SAHS in whom adenoidectomy/tonsillectomy is ineffective or not indicated. Mask discomfort, leak, skin rash, and noncompliance are the main factors associated with unsuccessful CPAP treatment. Tracheostomy is occasionally required in some children.

38. What is the obesity hypoventilation syndrome in children?

Obesity hypoventilation syndrome (OHS) is characterized by daytime hypercapnia, hypoxemia, and hypersomnolence in obese children without intrinsic pulmonary disease. Evidence indicates that severe SAHS is a contributing cause of OHS, with repeated episodes of nocturnal hypoxemia and hypercapnia resulting in attenuation of both the hypoxic and hypercapnic ventilatory drives during wakefulness, attenuation of ventilatory drive during sleep and poor chest wall compliance. Whether an obese child develops OHS probably depends on the interaction of the individual child's carbon dioxide response and the work of breathing. It is unclear whether the diminished ventilatory responsiveness precedes obesity or is acquired.

39. What is Pickwickian syndrome?

Pickwickian syndrome is another name for obesity hypoventilation syndrome. It originates from the fictional character Joe, "the fat boy" created by Charles Dickens in the *Pickwick Papers*. The term Pickwickian syndrome is often used loosely. If used at all, the term should be reserved for describing very obese patients with daytime sleepiness and elevated daytime pCO_2 without evidence of intrinsic pulmonary or neurologic disease.

40. What is Prader-Willi syndrome? How does it affect sleep?

The clinical phenotype of Prader-Willi syndrome consists of short stature, hypogonadism, developmental delay, and childhood onset of severe obesity. Up to 50% of boys with Prader-Willi syndrome develop obsessive behaviors related primarily to food, such as insatiable appetite and frequent foraging for food at night. One-third of children with Prader-Willi syndrome have sleep-onset REM periods and REM sleep during naps. These patients have decreased slow-wave sleep and poor sleep quality compared with normal patients. Up to 95% of children with Prader-Willi syndrome may have excessive daytime sleepiness. Some patients seem to benefit from daytime stimulant treatment, even after SAHS is adequately treated.

41. What causes Prader-Willi syndrome? How common is it?

The vast majority of cases of Prader-Willi syndrome are sporadic, caused by lack of the paternal segment 15q11 and resulting in failure to normally suppress certain genes on the maternal chromosome. This phenomenon is known as imprinting and is required for normal development. The frequency of Prader-Willi syndrome is estimated to be 1 in 25,000 births. It may be the most common known genetic cause of human obesity.

SCOLIOSIS AND NEUROMUSCULAR DISEASE

42. How does scoliosis interfere with normal ventilation during sleep?

Spinal deformity reduces chest wall compliance, thereby increasing the elastic force that the diaphragm must overcome to generate an adequate tidal volume. Scoliosis changes the position of the spine and lower ribs so that that length and configuration of the diaphragm becomes abnormal and its force of contraction is diminished. The diaphragm may also be intrinsically weak if the scoliosis is due to a neuromuscular disorder. These problems are compounded by reduced tone of the upper airway muscles during REM sleep. The upper airway narrows and becomes more collapsible when diaphragm contraction generates a negative pressure within the airway during inspiration. Biochemical respiratory drive in scoliosis is usually maintained unless the patient has severe sleep deprivation due to repeated arousals from apnea or chronic hypercapnia, which blunt the ventilatory response. Patients with severe kyphosis cannot increase ventilatory activity because of a combination of mechanical and chest deformity, airway distortion, and depressed ventilatory drive.

43. What are daytime indicators of sleep problems in children with scoliosis?

Nocturnal hypoventilation generally precedes respiratory failure, as diagnosed by conventional blood gas analysis during wakefulness. It may be detected even when waking blood gases are normal. Predicting when a child with severe scoliosis will proceed to nocturnal respiratory insufficiency is imprecise, but for the clinician the best indicators are the level and severity of the scoliosis measured by the Cobb angle, percent of predicted forced vital capacity (FVC), and the resting arterial pCO_2 during the day. Thoracic curves with Cobb angles as low as 80° have been associated with nocturnal ventilatory impairment. Patients with resting arterial $pCO_2 > 50$ mmHg should be carefully evaluated for nocturnal hypoventilation.

44. What are the signs and symptoms of sleep hypoventilation in children with neuromuscular disease?

Sleep hypoventilation may be recognized by clinical features such as morning headaches due to carbon dioxide retention and daytime sleepiness from sleep deprivation due to repeated apneas and arousals. Personality changes correlate with the degree of sleep deprivation rather than the abnormalities in arterial blood gases.

Nocturnal hypoxemia should be suspected in children with daytime hypercapnia or a decrease in supine FVC compared with upright FVC of more than 25%, which signals diaphragm weakness. Children with neuromuscular disease frequently have severe nocturnal hypoxemia, obstructive apneas, and hypoventilation. Respiratory failure at night is most severe in patients with the most abnormal daytime blood gases and probably occurs because respiratory muscle weakness and decreased compliance of the chest wall and lungs are common to both sleep and wakefulness. Loss of biochemical drive and reduction in respiratory muscle tone make ventilatory failure more severe in sleep. Mean oxygen saturation during both sleep and wakefulness probably determines when polycythemia and pulmonary hypertension develop. The greatest oxygen desaturation occurs in most patients during REM sleep. Coexisting lung disease and obesity contribute to sleep problems. The evaluation of a child with scoliosis suspected of having nocturnal hypoventilation includes an awake arterial blood gas in the supine position, upright and supine spirometry looking for a greater than 25% drop in FVC, and overnight polysomnographic study. The polysomnogram is the most accurate way to assess the severity of nocturnal oxygen desaturation, hypoventilation and sleep derangements.

45. Describe is the treatment of nocturnal hypoventilation in patients with scoliosis or neuromuscular disease.

Short-term ventilation has been associated with a marked improvement in clinical signs of respiratory failure in kyphoscoliosis. Patients have been provided noninvasive ventilatory support at night with negative pressure ventilators, nasal BiPAP or nasal intermittent positive pressure ventilation. For many children ventilatory support is initially required only at night to improve the quality of life and prognosis.

46. What sleeping problems occur in children with progressive neuromuscular diseases?

Nocturnal hypoventilation occurs in many children with progressive neuromuscular diseases such as Duchenne muscular dystrophy, spinal muscular atrophy, and congenital myopathies. Such children may benefit from use of noninvasive ventilation at night or may require tracheostomy and positive pressure ventilation. Sleep fragmentation, poor sleep continuity, and reduced REM and slow-wave sleep are commonly seen in older patients

BRAIN AND SPINAL DISORDERS

47. What sleep problems are associated with traumatic brain injuries in children?

Alterations in sleep patterns and sleep disturbances are a common manifestation of traumatic brain injury in children. In moderate-to-severe traumatic brain injuries, problems have been reported with the initiation and maintenance of sleep, alterations in sleep architecture, and excessive daytime sleepiness. SAHS and nocturnal alveolar hypoventilation have been reported after head trauma. In general, the greater the severity of the brain injury, the greater the effect of sleep maintenance problems on quality of life. Sleep disturbance may increase the intensity of other symptoms, such as fatigue, pain, and irritability. Sleep disorders may affect cognitive and behavioral functioning. Post-traumatic narcolepsy, delayed sleep phase disorder, post-traumatic hypersomnolence, and dreaming disturbances have been reported after traumatic brain injuries. Post-traumatic hypersomnolence can be a significant problem, leading to long-term disability in some patients.

48. What sleep problems are associated with spinal cord injuries?

Children with spinal cord injuries often complain of sleep maintenance problems and excessive daytime sleepiness. Sleep apnea with excessive daytime sleepiness has been reported in up to 40% of adults after spinal cord injury and is more common in complete motor injuries and quadriplegics. Pediatric studies are lacking, but clinical experience is similar.

49. What sleep problems are associated with spina bifida and Chiari type II malformations?

Children with spina bifida and Chiari type II malformations are at risk for central, obstructive, or mixed apneas during sleep. Some children require tracheostomy and mechanical ventilation due to severe central hypoventilation and/or upper airway obstruction.

CONGENITAL CENTRAL HYPOVENTILATION SYNDROME

50. What is congenital central hypoventilation syndrome?

The hallmark of congenital central hypoventilation syndrome (CCHS) is that affected infants cannot adequately ventilate during sleep. Some infants with the most severe forms have milder daytime hypoventilation, but most are normal while awake. The principal physiologic abnormality is insensitivity to hypercapnia. Hypoventilation occurs more severely or exclusively during sleep. The reduced central respiratory drive may be a complication of an earlier insult to the developing brain. Infants generally require tracheostomy and positive pressure ventilation. Some older children have been managed with nighttime negative pressure ventilation, mask positive pressure ventilation, or phrenic nerve stimulation.

51. During which stage of sleep do children with CCHS have their most abnormal breathing?

Unlike almost every other disorder, in which respiratory problems are worse in REM sleep, CCHS is associated with the worst impairment in ventilatory function during quiet sleep in infants or slow-wave sleep in older children.

52. What is Ondine's curse?

Ondine's curse was a popular diagnostic term until a few years ago for children with CCHS. The term is derived from a legened attributed to Greeks and Celtics that has various modern permutations. The legend, which combines elements of fantasy and tragedy, involves the unrequited love of a fairy/nymph for a knight. The key element, at least for pediatric pulmonologists, is a curse causing loss of the ability to breathe during sleep. In one version, the water nymph Ondine finds Sir Lawrence asleep in the arms of a rival and exclaims the immortal words, "As long as you are awake, you shall have your breath, but should you ever fall asleep, breath will be taken and you will die." The nymph appears in La Motte-Fouque's *Undine*, Giraudoux's *Ondine,* and Tchaikovsky's *Undine* (with some elements used in the ballet *Swan Lake*).

A sense of political correctness should encourage us to use the term CCHS since children, even naughty ones, should never really be cursed (although scolding may be sometimes necessary). In any case, the term as applied to CCHS is clearly a misnomer because the curse appears to be acquired rather than congenital!

53. What congenital comorbid conditions are common in children with CCHS?

The CCHS phenotype is associated with lower penetrance anomalies of the autonomic nervous system, including Hirschsprung's disease (aganglionosis of the colon) in up to 20% of infants and neural crest-derived tumors, such as ganglioneuromas and neuroblastomas. The term *neurocristopathy* describes the association of CCHS, congenital neuroblastoma, and Hirschsprung's disease.

54. Does CCHS have a genetic basis?

Yes. A genetic orgin of CCHS has long been suspected based on concordance in monozygotic twins, rare familial cases (siblings and mother-to-child transmission), and segregation analysis. Evidence suggests an autosomal dominant locus with low penetrance. Recently, heterozygous de novo mutations in the PHOX2B gene mapped to chromosome 4p12 were found in almost 60% of unrelated patients with CCHS, providing the strongest genetic link thus far.

DEPRESSION

55. What sleep problems are associated with childhood depression?

Depression in childhood is a problem of greater magnitude than generally appreciated. It is estimated that approximately 2% of children and up to 8% of adolescents suffer from major depression. Early studies of subjective sleep complaints in early-onset depression revealed that up to two-thirds of depressed children suffered from sleep-onset and sleep-maintenance insomnia. Half of children with endogenous type depression reported terminal insomnia, defined as early morning awakenings with an inability to return to sleep. Approximately 25% of adolescents with depression also complained of excessive daytime sleepiness. Of interest, approximately 10% of adolescents continued to experience insomnia after remission of depressive symptoms. Sleep complaints are the most prevalent symptom of major depression in adolescents

56. How do sleep characteristics of adolescents with depression compare with sleep characteristics of adults with depression?

Sleep structure in adolescents with depression resembles that seen in depressed adults, with reduced REM latency and prolonged sleep onset. Hospitalized psychotic and suicidal patients with depression have significantly longer sleep latencies and a trend toward reduced REM latency and increased REM time compared with outpatient, nonsuicidal control patients.

57. What is seasonal affective disorder? How prevalent is it in children?

Seasonal affective disorder (SAD) is defined as the occurrence of depressive episodes during at least two consecutive autumns and/or winters with remittance during the spring or summer and the absence of any other axis I psychiatric disorder. Surveys have revealed a prevalence rate of 3–4% in children. No gender differences in the prevalence of childhood seasonal mood changes have been noted.

58. How is seasonal affective disorder treated?

Double-blind, placebo-controlled trials of light therapy with 2 hours of dawn exposure plus 1 hour of bright-light therapy in the early evening in children with SAD appeared to be beneficial. Indeed, parental ratings showed a significant decrease in SAD symptoms during active treatment with light therapy compared with baseline, placebo, and washout periods. Increased awareness of primary care physicians of SAD should prompt early intervention with light therapy and possibly result in amelioration of SAD symptoms.

RELATED CONCERNS

59. What is sleep phase delay?

Sleep phase delay, commonly seen in teenagers, is the inability to fall asleep before midnight to 2:00 AM with a desire to awaken spontaneously at 10:00 AM to noon. It is a common cause of sleep-onset insomnia in adolescents. It may be associated with significant daytime fatigue, poor grades, and school absenteeism.

60. How common are nightmares in childhood?

Nightmares frequently occur in childhood. Up to 80% of children between the ages of 4 and 12 years report at least one occasional nightmare. However, frequent nightmares (> 1 per month) occur in only 15% of children. Nighttime fears are a common experience for most children. Up to 75% of children aged 4 to 12 years indicate that they have fears, most frequently of animals, fictitious characters such as witches or monsters, being kidnapped, and being teased by peers.

61. What sleep problems are seen in children with autism and pervasive developmental disorder?

Autism and pervasive developmental disorder (PDD) are defined as neuropsychiatric disorders characterized by a delay in the development of cognitive, social, and communicative skills with an onset during the first years of life. The estimated prevalence of autism is 1 per 1,000 children. To diagnose autism, a child must exhibit impairments in each of three domains: social relatedness, communication and play, and restricted interests and activities. Autism commonly occurs with other psychiatric and developmental disorders, including mental retardation, hyperactivity, anxiety, attentional problems, affective symptoms, and stereotypical or self-injurious behaviors.

Children with autism or PPD often present with extremely difficult sleep management problems, including severe sleep-onset and sleep-maintenance insomnia. They also may have increased periodic limb movements during sleep. Some children treated with psychotropic medications experience excessive weight gain, leading to obstructive apneas.

62. Why do children not wake up during fire alarms?

Children can be remarkably resistant to awakening by sound when asleep. Studies of auditory arousal thresholds during sleep have shown that the average stimulus required to elicit arousals is much higher in children than in adults. In one study, the frequency of awakenings was only 4.5% during slow-wave sleep, 34% during stage II sleep, and 50% during REM sleep, even at intensities up to 123 decibels (90–100 decibels above waking threshold levels). Normal speech is in the range of 40–60 decibels, jet engines are 125 decibels, and the danger of acoustic trauma is present at > 140 decibels.

Arousals from slow-wave sleep are very difficult to elicit and generally occur only with slow-wave sleep episodes after the first episode of REM sleep. Findings of enhanced sleep-sustaining processes during the first sleep cycle are expected because of a general absence of cortical or behavioral arousals associated with various parasomnias, such as sleepwalking, sleeptalking, and enuresis, that may occur during this time. The intensity of the sleep protective process is so overwhelming that it is virtually impossible to affect behavioral autonomic or EEG arousals during the first sleep cycle.

Despite some evidence that children may have improved capacity to awaken from sleep when confronted by their own name, the response to name largely, but not entirely, disappears in very deep sleep. The difficulty in awakening sleeping children with sound can lead to tragedy when children do not respond to home smoke detectors. This problem has created significant concerns in the home fire safety industry. The ability of smoke detectors to awaken children is currently under federal scrutiny.

63. When do infants develop EEG patterns typical for adult sleep?

Generally infants develop adult sleep patterns of sleep spindles and K complex (stage II sleep) by 4–5 months of age. By 6 months of age, 90% of infants have a greater amount of quiet sleep than REM sleep. By about 8 months of age REM sleep occupies about 30% of total sleep time, as in most adults.

BIBLIOGRAPHY

1. Amiel J, Laudier B, Attie–Bitach T, et al: Polyalanine expansion and frameshift mutations of the paired like homeobox gene PHOX2B in congenital central hypoventilation syndrome. Nature Genet 33:459–461, 2003.
2. Bandla H, Splaingard ML: Sleep problems in children with common medical disorders. Pediatr Clin North Am 51:203–227, 2004.
3. Sheldon S, Spire JP, Levy HB: Pediatric Sleep Medicine. Philadelphia, W.B. Saunders, 1992.

V. Miscellaneous Sleep Issues

26. FORENSIC SLEEP MEDICINE

Rosalind Cartwright, PhD

SLEEP-RELATED VIOLENCE

1. What forms of sleep-related violence have been recognized?

An episode of violence can arise out of a partial arousal from either rapid-eye-movement (REM) or non-REM (NREM) sleep. The attack behavior associated with either sleep stage may be against property, another person, or self. The episode may consist of a single punch or of acts as violent as rape, murder, or suicide.

2. Are different demographic characteristics associated with the two types?

REM-related violence, which is also called REM behavior disorder (RBD), is more often associated with the elderly, particularly those suffering from some neurodegenerative disorder. The NREM type, which is called sleepwalking violence or sometimes homicidal somnambulism, typically occurs first in late adolescence or young adulthood, and more frequently in males than females. People exhibiting RBD typically have no early childhood history of abnormal arousals from sleep, whereas people exhibiting sleepwalking violence have a strong personal and/or family history of prior sleepwalking, sleep terrors, or nocturnal enuresis.

3. What is the prevalence of sleepwalking violence?

Epidemiologic studies put the rate of self-reported current episodes of sleep-related violence at 2.1% in the general adult population. Most of these cases never come to the attention of a physician or sleep clinician or the courts, perhaps because the episodes are infrequent or mild in nature.

4. When sleepwalking violence results in bodily harm to another or in homicide, is the sleepwalker held responsible for his or her behavior?

The question of legal responsibility has been handled differently in different courts. The basic question is "What was the state of mind of the person at the time?" Was the person aware of the behavior and its consequences or not? Some people tried in British or Canadian courts have been acquitted under the ruling that such behaviors are "non-insane automatisms." The level of awareness at the time is often difficult to establish, particularly since one strong characteristic of this disorder is complete, or almost complete, amnesia for the event.

5. Is sleepwalking violence associated with a certain psychological profile?

Although profound remorse and depression are typical after an episode of violence, there is no specific prior psychopathology. Personality traits such as overcontrol of affect, internalization of anger, and a tendency to perfectionism have been noted in some cases in the forensic literature.

6. When does sleepwalking violence occur?

Most often sleepwalking violence occurs in the first third of the night's sleep—in the transition from slow-wave sleep before either the first or second REM period. No dream accompanies the behavior, as in RBD. The behavioral arousal may be into a sleepwalking state or have the characteristic panic-like behavior of a sleep terror or both, one following the other.

7. How does the person appear?

The eyes are open, and the person is able to orient well in space. However, the person does not recognize faces, even of loved ones, and typically does not respond to voices or to pain. The person may engage in complex motor behaviors such as driving or repairing a motorcycle. After an attack the person remains in a confused state for as long as an hour before full consciousness returns.

8. Why does sleepwalking violence occur?

An event is most likely to occur in a person who has the trait of genetic vulnerability to NREM parasomnia due to a strong family history in first-degree relatives and previous childhood episodes. When such a person is in a state of sleep deprivation, which is often secondary to a psychological stress for which the person has no ready solution, the stage is set for an increased likelihood of an episode.

9. Is a polysomnogram (PSG) helpful in making the diagnosis?

Yes, but not the traditional clinical study. Although it has been noted that a burst of hypersynchronous delta waves frequently precedes an abnormal arousal, this sign is not specific to sleepwalking violence, nor is it a reliable finding. The polysomnogram usually shows poor sleep efficiency with many interruptions of slow-wave sleep. However, this marked instability is also found in a number of other sleep disorders.

10. Should a special protocol be followed for the sleep study?

Three unique aspects need to be included in a proper diagnostic evaluation for sleep-related violence.

1. Because these studies may be court-ordered prior to a trial, the patient is likely to be in a highly anxious state and therefore not able to have a typical night of sleep. For this reason it is wise to plan to accommodate the patient to the laboratory by having one night of minimal recording, followed by a second night of recording with extra electroencephalography (EEG) leads to monitor for sleep architecture and possible seizure activity before a third diagnostic night.

2. Prior to the third night there should be a period of 36 hours of sleep deprivation.

3. The third, diagnostic night should be videotaped with good resolution because it may capture a behavioral arousal during the first third of the night. Extra-long leads should be used to allow the patient to get up without pulling off the leads.

11. If no behavioral arousal occurs, is the diagnosis ruled out?

No. According to new research, power density scoring reveals that delta power in the first cycle of sleepwalking patients is lower than that of age-matched controls. In addition, the delta power does not decrease across the night as is usual in normal sleepers.

12. Can an experimental stimulus be used to precipitate an event during PSG testing?

External stimuli, such as a tone, calling the patient by name, or touching the sleeper, have not usually been successful in provoking an episode in the laboratory. Often it appears that an internal stimulus is more successful. For example, an episode of apnea in a patient with sleep apnea has been reported to precipitate an abnormal arousal. Presumably any sleep disorder that is associated with repeated arousals from sleep, such as narcolepsy, might coexist with sleep-related violence. Other internal stimuli that have been implicated in triggering sleep-related violence include excessive caffeine use as well as some drugs and alcohol.

13. What factors in the patient's history are relevant in deciding the authenticity of sleepwalking violence when a legal case is involved?

Patients should be questioned about a history of previous parasomnia events. The one most clearly associated with adult sleep-related violence is a history of nocturnal enuresis (bedwetting past the age of 5 years). This is the parasomnia with the clearest evidence of a genetic component based on twin studies and family studies. Although the patient may not be able to supply a childhood history of sleepwalking or sleep terrors due to the profound amnesia for such events, they usually have some more memory of experiencing a wet bed on awakening. However, the sporadic nature of these events points to the importance of environmental or psychosocial factors as well as genetics.

14. If a child with sleepwalking, sleep terror, or enuresis is free of precipitating events in the teen-age years, is he or she past the age of vulnerability to sleepwalking violence?

No. Many patients have a period through the teen-age years in which they do not experience such events, only to have them return in a more severe form in adulthood.

15. Beside the PSG and history of previous episodes, what other data should be gathered and reviewed before reaching a diagnosis?

A psychiatric examination to rule out a dissociation disorder and alcohol or substance abuse history, a neurologic examination to rule out a seizure disorder, and psychological testing to investigate the patient's degree of impulse control help to fill in the picture. A lack of motivation for the attack on the victim and failure to cover it up are additional substantiating characteristics of sleepwalking violence. The police report of previous complaints or charges of violent behavior should also be taken into account.

16. What are the treatment options for sleepwalking violence? How successful are they?

To control the partial arousals in the first two sleep cycles, clonazepam has been highly successful in a dose range of 0.5 to 3 mg. To avoid sedation effects in the morning, clonazepam should be started at the lowest dose and increased slowly. Most patients can be controlled at less than the maximum dose without developing tolerance. There may be a problem in obtaining the medication if the person is convicted for the sleep-related violent attack. If the court rules that this defense is not credible, treatment may be denied. In any case, patients must learn to avoid sleep deprivation and to keep to a regular sleep-wake schedule. To avoid the increase in psychological distress, they need to learn and demonstrate mastery of stress management skills. This strategy is most important if no medication is ordered. Some sleepwalkers have been treated successfully with hypnosis, using the instruction that if their feet hit the floor, they will awaken fully. Hypnosis may not be sufficient to prevent an attack on a bed partner or cellmate.

17. Is it possible to predict a sleep-related violence attack?

Probably not—but an ounce of prevention may avoid a pound of trouble. All physicians should inquire about their patients' childhood history of sleepwalking, sleep terrors, and nocturnal enuresis. When the history is positive, the patient should be warned about the importance of good sleep hygiene, regular sleep hours, and the need to alert the physician if the patient experiences a period of stress leading to sleep loss so that the problem can be treated promptly.

18. Do we know why a nonpsychotic person should become abruptly physically or sexually aggressive without having formed any conscious intent and without memory of the attack?

The presumption is that some severe waking stress has mobilized strong basic survival drives of fight or flight or procreation. If these drives are constrained in sleep, they may be discharged safely in REM dreaming. However, in people with a genetic vulnerability to incomplete arousal during the transition from NREM to REM, these strong drives can precipitate a direct behavioral discharge that short-circuits the higher executive functions of the brain.

19. What research supports this model?

To date there is only one study in which a sleepwalking episode was recorded during a brain imaging study. This finding supports the concept that the brain is both partially asleep and partially awake, with reduced cortical parietal association area activity and an increase in thalamic cingulate circuits. Clearly this difficult area of research requires more attention.

20. What guidelines exist for providing expert witness testimony in such cases?

Most important is to be qualified by training and experience with similar cases. The expert should also be familiar with the diagnostic characteristics as outlined in the Diagnostic and Statistical Manual of the American Psychiatric Association for sleepwalking violence and the differential between this and similar disorders. The expert should not form an opinion until all data have been reviewed. It is also important to avoid a monetary incentive that might be presumed to influence the opinion. Fees should be reasonable and in line with the expert's usual hourly charge. The report should be open to review by peers.

BIBLIOGRAPHY

1. Hublin C, Kaprio J: Genetic aspects and genetic epidemiology of parasomnias. Sleep Med Rev 7:413–421, 2003.
2. Joncas S, Zarda A, Montplaisir J: The value of sleep deprivation as a diagnostic tool in adult sleepwalkers. Neurology 58:936–940, 2002.
3. Ohayon M, Caulet M, Priest R: Violent behavior during sleep. J Clin Psychiatry 58:369–376, 1997.
4. Schenck C, Mahowald M: Polysomnographically documented case of adult somnambulism with long distance automobile driving and frequent nocturnal violence: Parasomnia with continuing danger as a non-insane automatism? Sleep 18:765–772, 1995.
5. Schneck C, Mahowald M: Long-term nightly benzodiazepine treatment of injurious parasomnias and other disorders of disturbed nocturnal sleep in 170 adults. Am J Med 100:333–337, 1996.

APPENDIX: THE INTERNATIONAL CLASSIFICATION OF SLEEP DISORDERS REVISED 1997

1. Dyssomnias
   A. Intrinsic sleep disorders
      i. Psychophysiologic insomnia
      ii. Sleep state misperception
      iii. Idiopathic insomnia
      iv. Narcolepsy
      v. Recurrent hypersomnia
      vi. Idiopathic hypersomnia
      vii. Post-traumatic hypersomnia
      viii. Obstructive sleep apnea syndrome
      ix. Central sleep apnea syndrome
      x. Central alveolar hypoventilation syndrome
      xi. Periodic limb movement disorder
      xii. Restless legs syndrome
      xiii. Intrinsic sleep disorder NOS

   B. Extrinsic sleep disorders
      i. Inadequate sleep hygiene
      ii. Environmental sleep disorder
      iii. Altitude insomnia
      iv. Adjustment sleep disorder
      v. Insufficient sleep syndrome
      vi. Limit-setting sleep disorder
      vii. Sleep-onset association disorder
      viii. Food allergy insomnia
      ix. Nocturnal eating (drinking) syndrome
      x. Hypnotic-dependent sleep disorder
      xi. Stimulant-dependent sleep disorder
      xii. Alcohol-dependent sleep disorder
      xiii. Toxin-induced sleep disorder
      xiv. Extrinsic sleep disorder NOS

   C. Circadian-rhythm sleep disorders
      i. Time zone change (jet lag) syndrome
      ii. Shift work sleep disorder
      iii. Irregular sleep-wake pattern
      iv. Delayed sleep-phase syndrome
      v. Advanced sleep-phase syndrome
      vi. Non-24-hour sleep-wake disorder
      vii. Circadian rhythm sleep disorder NOS

2. Parasomnias
   A. Arousal disorder
      i. Confusional arousals
      ii. Sleepwalking
      iii. Sleep terrors

   B.   Sleep-wake transition disorders
       i.   Rhythmic movement disorder
      ii.   Sleep starts
     iii.   Sleep talking
     iv.   Nocturnal leg cramps

   C.   Parasomnias usually associated with REM sleep
       i.   Nightmares
      ii.   Sleep paralysis
     iii.   Impaired sleep-related penile erection
     iv.   Sleep-related painful painful erection
      v.   REM sleep-related sinus arrest
     vi.   REM sleep behavior disorder

   D.   Other parasomnias
       i.   Sleep bruxism
      ii.   Sleep enuresis
     iii.   Sleep-related abnormal swallowing syndrome
     iv.   Nocturnal paroxysmal dystonia
      v.   Sudden unexplained nocturnal death syndrome
     vi.   Primary snoring
    vii.   Infant sleep apnea
   viii.   Congenital central hypoventilation syndrome
     ix.   Sudden infant death syndrome
      x.   Benign neonatal sleep myoclonus
     xi.   Other parasomnia NOS

3.   Sleep disorders associated with mental, neurologic, or other medical disorders
   A.   Associated with mental disorders
       i.   Psychoses
      ii.   Mood disorders
     iii.   Anxiety disorders
     iv.   Panic disorders
      v.   Alcoholism

   B.   Associated with neurologic disorders
       i.   Cerebral degenerative disorders
      ii.   Dementia
     iii.   Parkinsonism
     iv.   Fatal familial insomnia
      v.   Sleep-related epilepsy
     vi.   Electrical status epilepticus of sleep
    vii.   Sleep-related headaches

   C.   Associated with other medical disorders
       i.   Sleeping sickness
      ii.   Nocturnal cardiac ischemia
     iii.   Chronic obstructive pulmonary disease
     iv.   Sleep-related asthma
      v.   Sleep-related gastroesophageal reflux
     vi.   Peptic ulcer disease
    vii.   Fibromyalgia

4.   Proposed sleep disorders
      i.   Short sleeper
      ii.   Long sleeper
      iii.   Subwakefulness syndrome
      iv.   Fragmentary myoclonus
      v.   Sleep hyperhidrosis
      vi.   Menstrual-associated sleep disorder
      vii.   Pregnancy-associated sleep disorder
      viii.   Terrifying hypnagogic hallucinations
      ix.   Sleep-related neurogenic tachypnea
      x.   Sleep-related laryngospasm
      xi.   Sleep choking syndrome

NOS indicates not otherwise specified.

Reprinted from American Sleep Disorders Association: International Classification of Sleep Disorders. Rochester, Minnesota, ASDA, 1997, with permission.

INDEX

Page numbers in **boldface type** indicate entire chapter.